# STUDY GUI

## TO THE
## AMERICAN PSYCHIATRIC PUBLISHING

# Textbook of
# Psychosomatic Medicine

# STUDY GUIDE

## TO THE

### AMERICAN PSYCHIATRIC PUBLISHING

# Textbook of Psychosomatic Medicine

### James A. Bourgeois, O.D., M.D.

Associate Professor of Clinical Psychiatry and Behavioral Sciences
Alan Stoudemire Professor of Psychosomatic Medicine
Director, Consultation-Liaison Service
University of California, Davis School of Medicine
Sacramento, California

### Robert E. Hales, M.D., M.B.A.

Joe P. Tupin Professor and Chair, Department of Psychiatry and Behavioral Sciences,
University of California, Davis, School of Medicine
Director, UC Davis Health System Behavioral Health Center
Director, UC Davis, Sierra Health Foundation MD/MBA Fellowship Program
Medical Director, Mental Health Services, County of Sacramento
Sacramento, California

### Narriman C. Shahrokh

Chief Administrative Officer, Department of Psychiatry and Behavioral Sciences
University of California, Davis School of Medicine
Sacramento, California

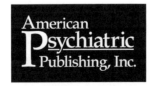

Washington, DC
London, England

Manufactured in the United States of America on acid-free paper
09  08  07  06  05    5  4  3  2

First Edition

Typeset in Revival BT and Adobe's The Mix

American Psychiatric Publishing, Inc.
1000 Wilson Boulevard
Arlington, VA 22209-3901
www.appi.org

# Contents

## Questions Only

## Answer Guide

Visit **www.appi.org** for more information about

*The American Psychiatric Publishing*

*Textbook of Psychosomatic Medicine.*

| | | |

Purchase the online version of this Study Guide at

**www.psychiatryonline.org**

and receive instant scoring and CME credits.

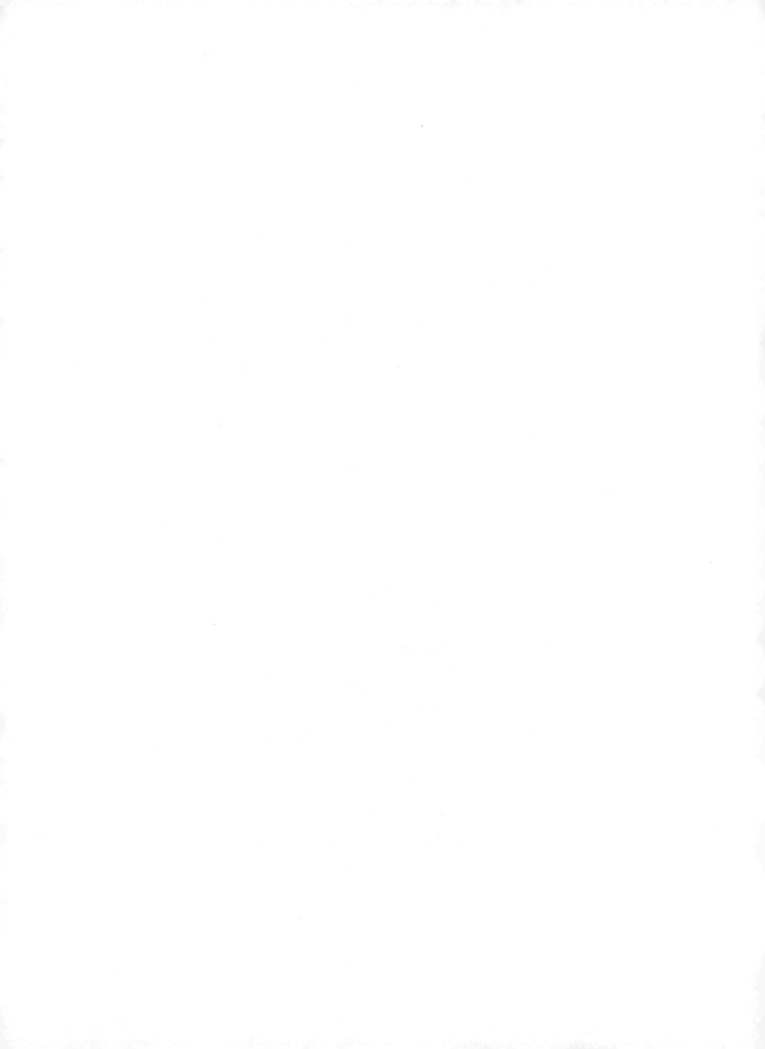

# C H A P T E R 1

# Psychiatric Assessment and Consultation

*Select the single best response for each question.*

1.1 Clinical assessment of memory and executive functions is an important component in the diagnosis and management of cognitive disorders. Regarding clinical assessment of cognitive function, all of the following are true *except*

A. Having the patient register and then later recall specific information (e.g., three objects) is a test of working memory.
B. Semantic memory is assessed by questions of general knowledge and naming of common objects.
C. Declarative memory includes both semantic and procedural memory components.
D. Having the patient name as many objects in a category (e.g., names of animals) as he or she can within 1 minute assesses frontal lobe function.
E. The go/no-go test of ability to inhibit a response assesses frontal lobe inhibitory function.

1.2 Language disorders involve the dominant cortical hemisphere and are important in neuropsychiatric illness encountered in psychosomatic medicine practice. Which of the following is *not* true regarding clinical presentation and assessment of the aphasias?

A. Naming of objects is affected in Broca's (expressive) aphasia.
B. Naming of objects is affected in Wernicke's (receptive) aphasia.
C. Wernicke's aphasia overlaps with psychotic disorders in that both conditions feature poor insight and incoherent speech.
D. Conduction aphasia features impaired naming with preserved repetition.
E. Global dysphasia combines features of both Broca's and Wernicke's aphasias.

1.3 In the task of differentiating primary psychiatric from secondary medical etiologies of hallucinatory experiences, the affected sensory modality may guide the clinician to the more likely etiology. Which of the following types of hallucinations is often seen in substance abuse?

A. Tactile.
B. Auditory.
C. Visual.
D. Gustatory.
E. Olfactory.

1.4    The adjunctive use of neuroimaging is an important part of psychosomatic medicine practice. The consultant often must determine which imaging modality is most appropriate for the clinical problem at hand. Which of the following pathological entities is better visualized by computed tomography (CT) than by magnetic resonance imaging (MRI)?

A.  Basal ganglia lesion (e.g., Parkinson's disease).
B.  Brain-stem lesion with motor signs.
C.  Cerebellar tumor.
D.  Acute intracranial hemorrhage.
E.  Vascular dementia with frontal lobe signs.

1.5    The electroencephalogram (EEG) may be a useful diagnostic tool in psychosomatic medicine, but it is subject to some important limitations. Which of the following clinical situations is most likely to be clarified by the use of an EEG?

A.  The search for a specific etiology of an established case of delirium.
B.  An insidious onset and slowly progressive dementia.
C.  Cognitive and motor deficits suggesting stroke.
D.  Distinguishing lingering delirium from schizophrenia in a psychotic patient.
E.  Localization of cerebral injury in traumatic brain injury.

1.6    Objective and validated standard test instruments have an adjunctive role in psychosomatic medicine, especially in the evaluation of suspected cognitive disorders. Which of the following statements is *true*?

A.  Because of the ubiquity of cognitive disorders in psychosomatic medicine, the consultant should evaluate every patient with a standardized cognitive assessment.
B.  The Folstein Mini-Mental State Examination (MMSE) is sensitive to subtle cognitive decline, even in premorbidly highly intelligent patients.
C.  The Mini-Cog combines a clock drawing task with a concentration task (serial subtractions or reverse spelling) from the MMSE.
D.  Clock drawing assesses temporoparietal and frontal cortical function.
E.  Formal cognitive testing results are valid even if the sensorium is clouded.

C H A P T E R    2

# Neuropsychological and Psychological Evaluation

*Select the single best response for each question.*

2.1    All of the following statements are true about battery-based approaches to neuropsychological testing *except*

    A.  They are highly standardized.
    B.  They may require special equipment.
    C.  They generally are more time-consuming than patient-centered approaches.
    D.  They provide a comprehensive assessment of cognitive function.
    E.  They are very sensitive to neurological dysfunction.

2.2    The Halstead-Reitan Neuropsychological Test Battery (HRNTB) consists of which of the following five types of measures?

    A.  Tests of verbal abilities.
    B.  Measures of spatial, sequential, and manipulatory abilities.
    C.  Tests of abstraction, reasoning, logical analysis, and concept formation.
    D.  All of the above.
    E.  None of the above.

2.3    Regarding the Minnesota Multiphasic Personality Inventory (MMPI), which of the following is *true*?

    A.  Many of the specific content scales are not sensitive to health concerns and neurological disorders.
    B.  An elevation in scores on scale 1 (Hypochondriasis) and scale 3 (Hysteria), with a significantly lower score on scale 2 (Depression), is referred to as the classic "conversion V" configuration.
    C.  Patients with seizure disorders, traumatic brain injury, or cardiovascular diseases have significantly lower scores on scale 1 (Hypochondriasis), scale 2 (Depression), and scale 3 (Hysteria).
    D.  Patients with rheumatoid arthritis often have elevated scores on scale 8 (Thought Disorder) and lower scores on scale 1 (Hypochondriasis) and scale 2 (Depression).
    E.  The presence of a conversion V proves the diagnosis of a somatoform disorder even without consideration of the patient's history, physical exam, or physical symptoms.

2.4    Which of the following is an example of a projective personality measure?

    A.  Minnesota Multiphasic Personality Inventory (MMPI).
    B.  Millon Clinical Multiaxial Inventory (MCMI).
    C.  Thematic Apperception Test (TAT).
    D.  Personality Assessment Inventory (PAI).
    E.  Millon Behavioral Health Inventory (MBHI).

2.5    Which of the following statements is *false*?

A.  Objective personality measures provide qualitative information on personality structure.
B.  Projective personality measures are time-consuming, sensitive to thought disorder, and provide rich psychodiagnostic information.
C.  Self-rating symptom scales are standardized, reliable, and valid for psychiatric diagnosis.
D.  Health-related quality-of-life scales are standardized, reliable, valid, and easily administered at bedside.
E.  Objective personality measures and projective personality measures are time-consuming (45–60 minutes) to complete.

# C H A P T E R   3

# Legal Issues

*Select the single best response for each question.*

3.1 The psychosomatic medicine specialist is often called upon to evaluate patients' ability to provide informed consent. All of the following are true regarding the doctrine of informed consent *except*

A. The *primary purpose* of the informed consent doctrine is to promote patient autonomy.

B. A *secondary purpose* of the informed consent doctrine is to facilitate rational decision making.

C. In emergency medical situations in which formal opportunity to provide consent is compromised, the law often "presumes" that consent is granted.

D. The determination of *emergency* is restricted to the patient's medical condition and not to availability of medical resources.

E. *Therapeutic privilege* is the exception to informed consent that is the least difficult to apply in practice.

3.2 Closely associated with clinical use of the informed consent doctrine is the determination of decisional capacity, in which the physician must render a decision regarding the patient's mental ability to appropriately participate in his or her own health care treatment. Which of the following is *true* of the psychiatrist's role in this clinical determination?

A. A psychiatrist at any level of training can declare a patient incompetent.

B. Only a board-certified psychiatrist can declare a patient incompetent.

C. Psychiatric illness is generally recognized by the law as rendering a patient incompetent even in the absence of cognitive impairment.

D. Adult patients are "presumed" competent unless they have been adjudicated incompetent or incapacitated by a medical illness.

E. The *Roe* case concluded that denial of illness was not grounds for a patient to be declared incompetent.

3.3 From their review of case law and scholarly literature, Appelbaum and colleagues (Appelbaum et al. 1987; Appelbaum and Grisso 1997) identified four key standards applied in the clinical determination of a patient's capacity to participate in health care decision making. Which of the following is *not* required to demonstrate decisional capacity?

A. Ability to communicate a choice regarding treatment.

B. Understanding of the treatment options available.

C. Formal cognitive testing revealing an "unimpaired" range of performance.

D. Appreciation of available diagnostic and therapeutic options.

E. Demonstration of rational decision making.

3.4 General incompetence (as defined by the Uniform Guardianship and Protective Proceedings Act [UGPPA]) may encompass impairment from numerous causes. Which of the following is *not* considered grounds for a determination of incompetence according to this act?

A. Minority status (age).
B. Psychiatric illness.
C. Advanced age.
D. Drug intoxication or chronic use.
E. Mental deficiency.

3.5 Regarding the *Cruzan* decision and its subsequent implications, which of the following statements is *true*?

A. The court ruled that the state could not prohibit the removal of a feeding tube in a comatose patient.
B. The state has an interest in the preservation of life, but not against the wishes of the parents of a comatose patient.
C. Physicians must seek clear and competent instructions from patients regarding foreseeable treatment decisions.
D. Decisions regarding future treatment require a durable power of attorney.
E. All states have subsequently enacted legislation empowering surrogate decision makers.

3.6 Advance directives are an increasingly important part of modern medical practice. All of the following are true *except*

A. Health care organizations are required to inform patients of their right to advance directives.
B. Health care organizations must inquire if patients have advance directives.
C. A copy of the advance directive may be added to the official medical record.
D. Federal law specifies the right to formulate an advance directive.
E. All 50 states allow for the writing of a durable power of attorney for health care decisions.

3.7 The psychosomatic medicine physician may be called upon to evaluate a patient who has requested an "against medical advice" (AMA) discharge. All of the following are true regarding AMA discharge requests *except*

A. The AMA form must be signed by the patient before the psychiatrist is called to evaluate.
B. Failures in physician–patient communication are common in AMA discharge situations.
C. External pressures (e.g., family responsibilities) often lead patients to request AMA discharge.
D. Many AMA discharge–requesting patients have addictive disorders that have not been adequately diagnosed or treated in the hospital.
E. The psychiatrist must evaluate danger to self or others as well as cognitive capacity for the AMA decision itself.

# C H A P T E R  4

# Ethical Issues

*Select the single best response for each question.*

4.1    The leading conception of the principles of biomedical ethics includes all of the following *except*

    A.  Respect for patient autonomy.
    B.  Beneficence.
    C.  Honesty.
    D.  Nonmaleficence.
    E.  Justice.


4.2    You are called to provide a psychiatric consultation on a man hospitalized on the oncology service in a general hospital. The two key questions you should attempt to answer are

    A.  Does this patient have a medical or psychiatric disorder that compromises his capacity to understand, appreciate, and reason with respect to the details of a given diagnostic or therapeutic procedure?
    B.  Is this patient able to appreciate the differences between clinical care and clinical research with regard to the treatment options being recommended by the oncologist?
    C.  On the basis of your clinical assessment, should this patient be allowed to give or refuse permission for medical care?
    D.  A and B.
    E.  A and C.


4.3    Which of the following sequences states the correct order of the continuum of decision-making capacity, from incapacitated to fully capacitated?

    A.  Able to assign a substitute decision maker → unable to make decisions → able to make medical decisions → able to appreciate the differences between clinical care and clinical research → fully capacitated.
    B.  Unable to make decisions → able to make medical decisions → able to assign a substitute decision maker → able to appreciate the difference between clinical care and clinical research → fully capacitated.
    C.  Unable to make decisions → able to assign a substitute decision maker → able to make medical decisions → able to appreciate the differences between clinical care and clinical research → fully capacitated.
    D.  Unable to make decisions → able to appreciate the differences between clinical care and clinical research → able to make medical decisions → able to assign a substitute decision maker → fully capacitated.
    E.  Able to assign a substitute decision maker → able to make medical decisions → unable to make decisions → able to appreciate the differences between clinical care and clinical research → fully capacitated.

4.4    Regarding medical decision making, which of the following statements is *true*?

   A. The parents of a disabled adult automatically remain the patient's legal guardians after their child's 18th birthday.
   B. Studies have found that most (75%–80%) individuals fill out an advance directive for health care when given the opportunity to do so.
   C. When an unmarried, incapacitated patient has an adult child, that adult child automatically is given medical decision making for the patient.
   D. The completion of an advance directive for health care allows patients to specify in writing the medical care they wish to receive under various catastrophic medical conditions.
   E. Substitute decision makers tend to base their decisions on what the patient would have wanted and not on what they themselves would have wanted had they been in the patient's place.


4.5    Regarding the effect of major depression on medically ill patients, which of the following statements is *false*?

   A. Major depression in medically ill patients often makes them decisionally incapacitated.
   B. Untreated depression has been linked to poor compliance with medical care.
   C. Depression produces more subtle distortions of decision making than does delirium or psychosis.
   D. Refusal of life-saving treatment by a depressed patient cannot be assumed to constitute lack of capacity.
   E. None of the above.

# C H A P T E R  5

# Psychological Responses to Illness

*Select the single best response for each question.*

5.1    In "Personality Types in Medical Management," Kahana and Bibring (1964) cited seven
       personality types that overlap with DSM-IV-TR (American Psychiatric Association 2000)
       personality disorders. In regard to these personality types, which of the following statements is
       *true?*

   A.  Dependent patients tend to adhere to treatment recommendations and have good frustration
       tolerance.
   B.  Obsessional patients have high control and information needs and rarely exhibit conflicts
       between compliance and defiance.
   C.  Histrionic patients should be required to directly confront their use of denial.
   D.  Masochistic patients should be managed by reassurance rather than by acknowledgement of
       their chronic sense of suffering.
   E.  Narcissistic patients' sense of entitlement should be reframed rather than being either
       directly reinforced or challenged.

5.2    The physician's countertransference response to patients is a crucial source of clinical data, both
       for understanding patients and for physician self-monitoring. Which of the following "personality
       type–countertransference response" pairings is *correct?*

   A.  Dependent: feeling erotic attraction to patient.
   B.  Obsessional: feeling little sense of connection to patient, finding it difficult to engage with
       patient.
   C.  Histrionic: feeling powerful and/or needed.
   D.  Masochistic: feeling angry, frustrated, helpless.
   E.  Narcissistic: feeling overwhelmed, trying to avoid patient.

5.3    Folkman et al. (1986) identified eight categories of coping styles in a factor analysis of the Ways
       of Coping Questionnaire–Revised. A patient who acknowledges a personal role in a problematic
       situation exemplifies which of the following?

   A.  Confrontative coping.
   B.  Accepting responsibility.
   C.  Distancing.
   D.  Self-controlling.
   E.  Planful problem solving.

5.4   Vaillant (1993) proposed a hierarchy of defense mechanisms ranked according to degree of adaptivity. Which of the following sequences (from a low to a high degree of adaptivity) is correct?

A.  Psychotic, narcissistic, neurotic, mature.
B.  Immature/borderline, neurotic, mature, adaptive.
C.  Psychotic, immature/borderline, neurotic, mature.
D.  Immature/borderline, narcissistic, neurotic, adaptive.
E.  Immature/borderline, narcissistic, neurotic, mature.


5.5   In Vaillant's (1993) hierarchy of defense mechanisms, a patient with a serious illness who consciously puts the illness "out of mind" is using which of the following defenses?

A.  Suppression.
B.  Repression.
C.  Sublimation.
D.  Displacement.
E.  Intellectualization.


5.6   *Denial* is an important and highly nuanced concept in illness and adaptation. Research has shown various effects of denial on physical outcomes. Which of the following statements is *true*?

A.  According to Hackett and Cassem (1974), myocardial infarction (MI) patients who were "minor deniers" had better clinical outcomes than "major deniers."
B.  According to Levenson et al. (1989), among angina patients, "low deniers" had better clinical outcomes than "high deniers."
C.  Among patients awaiting heart transplantation studied by Young et al. (1991), denial was associated with a worse survival rate.
D.  According to Levine et al. (1987), "major deniers" had shorter intensive care unit (ICU) stays but higher rates of noncompliance.
E.  According to Fricchione et al. (1992), increased denial was associated with more mood symptoms and sleep disturbance in renal disease patients.


5.7   Although anger is a common response to the threat of serious illness, anger in a patient often presents significant countertransference challenges for the physician. Significant anger under stress, such as when a clinical diagnosis remains unclear, is likely to be expressed by patients with all of the following personality disorders *except*

A.  Obsessive-compulsive.
B.  Paranoid.
C.  Narcissistic.
D.  Borderline.
E.  Antisocial.

# C H A P T E R  6

# Delirium

*Select the single best response for each question.*

6.1    Regarding the altered affect frequently observed in patients with delirium, which of the following statements is *false*?

    A.  Increased irritability is common.
    B.  Affect is related to the mood preceding the delirium.
    C.  Lability is common.
    D.  Affect is usually incongruent with context.
    E.  Hypoactive delirium is often mislabeled as depression.

6.2    Regarding the epidemiology of delirium, which of the following statements is *true*?

    A.  The elderly are at higher risk of developing delirium than are younger adults.
    B.  Children and adolescents are at higher risk of developing delirium than are adults.
    C.  Up to 60% of nursing home patients older than 65 years may have delirium.
    D.  All of the above.
    E.  A and C.

6.3    Which of the following symptoms, tests, or treatments can distinguish hyperactive from hypoactive delirium?

    A.  The electroencephalogram (EEG) shows diffuse slowing for hyperactive delirium and diffuse increased activity for hypoactive delirium.
    B.  Patients with hyperactive delirium are responsive to neuroleptics, whereas patients with hypoactive delirium are not.
    C.  Patients with hyperactive delirium have selective cognitive deficits, whereas patients with hypoactive delirium have diffuse cognitive deficits.
    D.  Patients with hyperactive delirium have higher mortality rates, whereas patients with hypoactive delirium have lower mortality rates.
    E.  Delirium due to drug-related causes is most commonly hyperactive, whereas delirium due to metabolic disturbances is more frequently hypoactive.

6.4    Regarding delirium assessment instruments, which of the following statements is *true?*

   A.  The Confusion Assessment Method (CAM) is based on DSM-III-R (American Psychiatric Association 1987) criteria and is intended for use by nonpsychiatric clinicians in a hospital setting.
   B.  The Delirium Rating Scale (DRS) has two forms—a full-scale 11-item form and a 4-item form.
   C.  The Memorial Delirium Assessment Scale (MDAS) is a 10-item scale assessing a breadth of delirium features and can function both to clarify diagnosis and to assess symptom severity because of its hierarchical nature.
   D.  The delirium assessment tool most commonly used by nurses is the Delirium Rating Scale—Revised–98 (DRS-R-98), a 30-point scale with cutoffs for levels of confusion severity.
   E.  The Organic Brain Syndrome Scale is based on DSM-IV (American Psychiatric Association 1994) criteria and includes 16 items, with 3 diagnostic items separable from 13 severity items that form a severity scale.


6.5    The EEG finding most typically seen in patients with delirium is

   A.  Low-voltage fast activity.
   B.  Diffuse slowing.
   C.  Frontocentral spikes.
   D.  Delta bursts.
   E.  None of the above.


6.6    The best-established neurotransmitter alteration in delirium is

   A.  Increased dopaminergic activity.
   B.  Increased cholinergic activity.
   C.  Increased gamma-aminobutyric acid (GABA)ergic activity.
   D.  Decreased serotonergic activity.
   E.  Decreased cholinergic activity.

# CHAPTER 7

# Dementia

*Select the single best response for each question.*

7.1     The distinction of cortical versus subcortical dementia provides a clinically useful framework for classification of clinical symptoms and dementia syndromes. Among the following neurodegenerative disorders that lead to dementia, which one most typically results in cortical dementia?

    A.  Dementia with Lewy bodies.
    B.  Parkinson's disease.
    C.  Huntington's disease.
    D.  Wilson's disease.
    E.  Progressive supranuclear palsy.

7.2     In dementia of the Alzheimer's type (DAT), numerous putatively protective factors have been proposed. Which of the following proposed protective factors is considered confirmed?

    A.  Low cholesterol.
    B.  Apolipoprotein ε3 allele.
    C.  Apolipoprotein ε2 allele.
    D.  Statin drugs.
    E.  Vitamin E.

7.3     In vascular dementia, numerous risk factors have been identified that roughly parallel the risk for coronary artery disease. Which of the following vascular dementia risk factors is considered confirmed?

    A.  Atrial fibrillation.
    B.  Hypertension.
    C.  Excess alcohol use.
    D.  Hyperlipidemia.
    E.  Female sex.

7.4     Cortical dementia (of which dementia of the Alzheimer's type is the prototype) can be identified by a common constellation of specific cognitive symptoms. All of the following symptoms are consistent with cortical dementia *except*

    A.  Apathy leading to akinetic mutism.
    B.  Amnesia which is not helped by cueing.
    C.  Aphasia.
    D.  Apraxia.
    E.  Agnosia.

7.5   The distinction of cortical versus subcortical dementia on clinical grounds may be an important differentiation in clinical practice. Which of the following clinical findings is more consistent with subcortical than with cortical dementia?

A.  Normal gait.
B.  Loss of initiative.
C.  Less frequent mood symptoms.
D.  Pathological reflexes.
E.  Absence of extrapyramidal side effects (EPS).


7.6   In frontotemporal dementia, all of the following symptoms or signs are typical *except*

A.  Irritability.
B.  Decreases in social judgment.
C.  Decreased impulse control with acting out.
D.  Early cognitive impairment.
E.  Hyperorality.


7.7   Prognosis in dementia of the Alzheimer's type is an important aspect of clinical care for these patients. Which of the following statements is *true*?

A.  Progression of deterioration is usually 4–6 Mini-Mental State Examination (MMSE) points per year.
B.  Cognitive deterioration is more rapid if Lewy bodies are absent.
C.  Psychotic symptoms at baseline portend more rapid decline.
D.  Delusions and/or hallucinations are more persistent than agitation and depression as the disease progresses.
E.  Basic activities of daily living (ADLs) are more seriously impaired than are instrumental ADLs.


7.8   Among the following medications, which antipsychotic agent would be preferred in Parkinson's disease or Lewy body dementia presenting with psychosis and agitation?

A.  Haloperidol.
B.  Chlorpromazine.
C.  Risperidone.
D.  Clozapine.
E.  Thioridazine.

# C H A P T E R   8

# Aggression and Violence

*Select the single best response for each question.*

8.1    Which of the following characteristics are usually *not* indicative of impulsive aggression?

    A.  Unplanned.
    B.  Explosive.
    C.  Deliberate.
    D.  All of the above.
    E.  None of the above.

8.2    Which of the following statements concerning aggression is *true*?

    A.  Aggression and violence in inpatient settings appear to be relatively frequent in the 24 hours immediately prior to discharge.
    B.  Involuntary admission rarely precipitates aggressive acts and violence.
    C.  Substance users may become aggressive soon after admission.
    D.  A rapid increase in the risk of aggression in patients with schizophrenia within a few days after admission is common.
    E.  Patient–staff conflicts, such as the denial of privileges, rarely precipitates aggression.

8.3    The neurotransmitter system(s) involved in the modulation of aggression include

    A.  Serotonin.
    B.  Norepinephrine.
    C.  Dopamine.
    D.  All of the above.
    E.  None of the above.

8.4    The diagnostic term *intermittent explosive disorder*

    A.  Refers to recurrent episodes of explosive anger not explained by psychosis or some other mental disorder.
    B.  Has been used to describe rage attacks in association with lesions of the hypothalamus and amygdala.
    C.  Has been used as a label for males with a history of conduct disorder.
    D.  May be applied to individuals with antisocial personality disorder who exhibit uncontrollable rage.
    E.  Can be used as an additional diagnosis for individuals with attention-deficit/hyperactivity disorder (ADHD) who show symptoms of explosive anger.

8.5 Effective de-escalation techniques for controlling and terminating mild to moderate aggression in hospital settings include all of the following *except*

A. Maintain a safe distance.
B. Avoid sudden movements.
C. Avoid personalizing yourself.
D. Stay at the same height as the patient.
E. Do not touch the patient.

# C H A P T E R   9

# Depression

*Select the single best response for each question.*

9.1 Depression rating scales may be helpful to the clinician in detecting mood symptoms in medically ill patients. Which of the following statements is *true*?

   A. The Center for Epidemiologic Studies Depression Scale (CES-D) is a 20-item scale validated for use in the medically ill.
   B. The Hospital Anxiety and Depression Scale (HADS) is useful in medically ill populations because it assesses many somatic symptoms of depression.
   C. The Beck Depression Inventory–II (BDI-II) is only moderately valid in medically ill patients, because it addresses few somatic symptoms.
   D. The Patient Health Questionnaire (PHQ) requires clinician administration.
   E. The HADS has better sensitivity and specificity for depression in medical illness than does the PHQ.

9.2 The interrelationship between coronary artery disease (CAD) and depression is complex but clinically important to psychosomatic medicine practice. All of the following are true *except*

   A. Depression increases morbidity and mortality risk in CAD.
   B. The American College of Cardiology regards depression as a primary risk factor for CAD.
   C. CAD patients with depression have an increased neuroendocrine response to stress.
   D. The Sertraline Antidepressant Heart Attack Trial (SADHART) found only modest effects of sertraline on cardiac function.
   E. The Enhancing Recovery in Coronary Heart Disease (ENRICHD) study, which used cognitive-behavioral therapy (CBT) and selective serotonin reuptake inhibitors (SSRIs), found no decrease in recurrent myocardial infarction (MI) risk with these interventions.

9.3 The relationship between depression and cancer is also important in psychosomatic medicine. Many specific cancer sites are associated with a notably higher risk for depression. Which of the following is *not* generally associated with a significantly higher risk for depression?

   A. Lung cancer.
   B. Pancreatic cancer.
   C. Central nervous system (CNS) cancer.
   D. Oropharyngeal cancer.
   E. Skin cancer.

9.4    Depression and neurological disease are commonly comorbid. All of the following statements are true regarding depression in neurological disease *except*

A. The Beck Depression Inventory (BDI) is not useful in the assessment of depression in Parkinson's disease, because the physical symptoms of Parkinson's disease affect the interpretation of the BDI.
B. Depression in Parkinson's disease is a major determinant of quality of life, more so than the severity of the motor impairment or the effects of medications.
C. Poststroke depression increases the mortality rate at 1 year after stroke.
D. Late-life-onset depression and "depressive pseudodementia" confer an increased risk of eventual diagnosis of dementia of the Alzheimer's type.
E. Dementia of the Alzheimer's type, when complicated by depression, is associated with an increased rate of nursing home placement, decline in activities of daily living (ADLs), and cognitive decline.


9.5    Selective serotonin reuptake inhibitors (SSRIs) are useful for treatment of major depression in the medically ill. Controlled trials have demonstrated benefit of SSRIs for depression in all of the following illnesses *except*

A. Cardiac disease.
B. Stroke.
C. Cancer.
D. HIV.
E. Parkinson's disease.


9.6    Which of the following novel antidepressants is *most* likely to rapidly alleviate insomnia and anorexia in cancer patients?

A  Moclobemide.
B. Venlafaxine.
C. Bupropion.
D. Mirtazapine.
E. Nefazodone.

# C H A P T E R   1 0

# Suicidality

*Select the single best response for each question.*

10.1    Which of the following statements concerning completed suicide is *true*?

    A. The known suicide rate in 2001 was twice as high as it was in 1900.
    B. Between 1990 and 2001, suicide rates increased in every age category.
    C. In 2001, annual suicide rates per 100,000 individuals increased throughout the life span from childhood to old age.
    D. The suicide rate among women is three times higher than that among men.
    E. In 2001, white Americans killed themselves at less than half the rate of nonwhite Americans.

10.2    In general, patients who attempted suicide, in comparison with those who died by suicide,

    A. Did not have long-standing mental illness.
    B. Did not have carefully considered plans.
    C. Did not have command hallucinations.
    D. Were not ruminative about their suicide intent.
    E. All of the above.

10.3    It has been repeatedly shown in general-population studies conducted in the United States and Europe that the vast majority of completed suicides are associated with

    A. Depression.
    B. Schizophrenia.
    C. Alcoholism.
    D. A and C.
    E. A and B.

10.4    Which of the following statements concerning suicide in medically ill patients is *false*?

    A. The majority of terminally ill cancer patients have a high desire for hastened death.
    B. Suicides in the medically ill appear to be related to unrecognized comorbid psychiatric illnesses.
    C. The will to live in terminally ill patients may be best predicted by presence and severity of depression; anxiety; shortness of breath; and sense of well-being.
    D. Cancer patients who die by suicide are psychiatrically similar to noncancer patients who commit suicide.
    E. Most patients who decide to stop dialysis are not influenced by major depression or suicidal ideation.

10.5 With regard to physician-assisted suicide, the United States Supreme Court in 1997 ruled that

A. There is a constitutional right to physician-assisted suicide.
B. States can prohibit physician conduct in which the primary purpose is to hasten death.
C. States cannot enact legislation that allows physician-assisted suicide.
D. All of the above.
E. None of the above.

# C H A P T E R   1 1

# Mania, Catatonia, and Psychosis

*Select the single best response for each question.*

11.1 It may be difficult to differentiate secondary mania from delirium in the acutely ill patient, because many of the presenting symptoms overlap. Which of the following symptoms is more suggestive of secondary mania than of delirium?

A. Waxing and waning course.
B. Variable level of consciousness.
C. Visual hallucinations.
D. Pressured speech.
E. Visual illusions.

11.2 Secondary mania may be either transient or relatively persistent, depending in substantial part on the putative etiological agent or condition. Which of the following would more likely be associated with transient/reversible rather than persistent secondary mania?

A. Traumatic brain injury.
B. Stroke.
C. Dopamine agonists.
D. Neoplasm.
E. Multiple sclerosis.

11.3 Endocrine disturbances and substances of abuse are associated with secondary mania. All of the following statements are true *except*

A. Hyperthyroidism may cause mania.
B. Hypothyroidism may cause mania.
C. Depression is more common following systemic use of corticosteroids than is mania.
D. Psychotic symptoms have been reported in 50% of hypomanic or depressive episodes following corticosteroid use.
E. Hypothyroidism induces rapid cycling in established bipolar disorder patients.

11.4 Core features of catatonia include all of the following symptoms or signs *except*

A. Stupor.
B. Motoric immobility.
C. Mutism.
D. Catalepsy.
E. Auditory hallucinations.

11.5 Patients with seizure disorders commonly have comorbid psychiatric illness. Notably, psychotic symptoms are a significant problem that may complicate diagnosis and management. All of the following are true *except*

A. Psychotic symptoms are most common during the interictal phase.
B. Psychotic symptoms are most common with evidence of left-sided seizure foci or temporal lobe lesions.
C. Psychotic symptoms associated with nonconvulsive status epilepticus are more common with partial complex seizures.
D. Postictal psychotic symptoms typically occur immediately following a seizure.
E. Postictal psychosis follows an increase in seizure frequency.

11.6 Psychotic symptoms may occur in patients with kidney disease and require treatment. Which of the following antipsychotics require dosage modification when used in patients with renal failure?

A. Ziprasidone.
B. Olanzapine.
C. Haloperidol.
D. Clozapine.
E. Risperidone.

# Anxiety Disorders

*Select the single best response for each question.*

12.1   A recent meta-analysis identified five variables that correlate with higher rates of panic disorder among individuals seeking treatment for chest pain in emergency rooms. All of the following variables were identified *except*

    A.  Absence of coronary artery disease.
    B.  Atypical quality of chest pain.
    C.  Male gender.
    D.  Younger age.
    E.  High level of self-reported anxiety.

12.2   A life-threatening illness, such as cancer, is a stressor that can precipitate posttraumatic stress disorder (PTSD). However, this trauma is different from more usual PTSD stressors in which of the following ways?

    A.  The threat is external.
    B.  The principal stressor relates to the fear of recurrence.
    C.  The ongoing stressor is the memory of past events.
    D.  The threat arises from one's own body.
    E.  B and D.

12.3   Regarding therapies that have been found effective in reducing anxiety and physical symptoms in medically ill patients, which of the following statements is *false*?

    A.  Muscular conditions such as tension headaches respond better to more cognitive techniques.
    B.  Migraine headaches respond better to autogenic training.
    C.  Relaxation techniques have been used to reduce pain in patients with chronic pain.
    D.  Guided imagery with relaxation has been shown to be an effective technique for reducing anxiety.
    E.  Musculoskeletal disorders may respond better to muscle relaxation.

12.4   Advantages of selective serotonin reuptake inhibitors (SSRIs) in treating anxiety disorders in medically ill patients include all of the following *except*

    A.  SSRIs do not produce cardiac conduction problems.
    B.  SSRIs do not cause orthostatic hypotension.
    C.  SSRIs do not lead to physical dependence.
    D.  SSRIs do not produce sexual dysfunction.
    E.  SSRIs have few side effects.

12.5    Regarding the use of beta-adrenergic blockers to treat anxiety symptoms, which of the following statements is *true*?

A. Beta-blockers are most efficacious in treating panic disorder.
B. Beta-blockers work best when used in specific anxiety-producing situations.
C. Beta-blockers are the treatment of choice for anxiety in chronic obstructive pulmonary disease (COPD) patients.
D. Patients with insulin-dependent diabetes should be prescribed nonselective beta-blockers.
E. Beta-blockers can improve peripheral vascular disease.

# CHAPTER 13

# Somatization and Somatoform Disorders

*Select the single best response for each question.*

13.1   The more general concept of somatization (bridging several of the somatoform disorders) may be used as an explanatory model for many behaviors presenting in the physically ill patient. Which of the following statements is *true*?

A.  Somatization is best understood as a defense against the acknowledgment of a psychiatric disorder.

B.  Fifty percent or more of depressed patients in primary care clinics manifest predominantly somatic complaints.

C.  Somatic symptoms in depression are related to mood symptoms alone, not to concurrent anxiety.

D.  Although somatization is common in panic disorder, hypochondriacal fears of a specific illness are not.

E.  Somatization in schizophrenia is unrelated to high levels of "expressed emotion" in family members.

13.2   Various pathophysiological mechanisms have been employed to provide explanatory models for somatization. These include several physiological, psychological, and interpersonal mechanisms. Which of the following would be considered a physiological (as opposed to a psychological) mechanism?

A.  Cerebral information processing.

B.  Perceptual factors.

C.  Beliefs.

D.  Mood.

E.  Personality factors.

13.3   The clinical management of somatization is best accomplished along several dimensions, and the psychosomatic medicine consultant may be of help to colleagues in effectuating such management plans. Three possible management approaches—reattribution, psychotherapeutic, and directive—to the patient with somatization disorder have been described. All of the following are true *except*

A.  The reattribution approach seeks to link physical symptoms to psychological factors in the patient's life.

B.  The psychotherapeutic approach focuses on the centrality of the relationship between patient and physician.

C.  The directive approach frames the somatization behavior as a medical problem, and interventions are made in a medical context.

D. The psychotherapeutic approach is preferred for openly hostile patients who deny psychological factors in their symptoms.

E. The reattribution approach is useful in medical inpatient settings with reasonably insightful patients.

13.4    In regard to the clinical features of somatization disorder, all of the following are true *except*

A. Symptoms begin before the age of 30 years, often during the teens.

B. Depression, substance abuse, and antisocial personality disorder are common in first-degree relatives of somatization disorder patients.

C. Women with somatization disorder are less likely to have a history of sexual abuse than are women with primary major depression.

D. Patients present their histories in a vague yet dramatic and colorful manner.

E. The majority of somatization disorder patients have psychiatric comorbidity.

13.5    Which of the following is *not* among the most common comorbid psychiatric conditions in somatization disorder?

A. Obsessive-compulsive disorder.

B. Major depression.

C. Dysthymic disorder.

D. Panic disorder.

E. Simple phobia.

13.6    Conversion disorder is a somatoform disorder that often has an acute and dramatic presentation. Which of the following is *not* true of conversion disorder?

A. Presentations include pseudoseizures, ataxia, and sensory deficits.

B. Social settings with substantial secondary gain increase the likelihood of conversion disorder.

C. A relationship with childhood abuse is especially common in pseudoseizure conversion patients.

D. Higher rates of conversion disorder are found in highly developed nations.

E. The paradoxical emotional response of *la belle indifference* does not confer prognostic significance.

13.7    Patients with hypochondriasis can lead a physician to pursue an extensive diagnostic workup. Which of the following statements is *true*?

A. Onset of hypochondriasis is most common in middle or late middle age.

B. Hypochondriasis patients accept that good health can involve minor symptoms.

C. Psychiatric comorbidity in hypochondriasis includes generalized anxiety disorder, major depression, and panic disorder.

D. Because of their fear of "legitimate" medical illness, patients with hypochondriasis are unlikely to use alternative health care practices.

E. Presence of a "real" comorbid medical illness is associated with a worse prognosis.

# C H A P T E R  1 4

# Deception Syndromes: Factitious Disorders and Malingering

*Select the single best response for each question.*

14.1    Regarding simulated physical diseases, which of the following statements are *true*?

A.  Somatoform disorders are considered to be of unconscious etiology.
B.  Factitious disorders are considered to be of conscious production and unconscious motivation.
C.  Malingering is considered to be of conscious production and motivation.
D.  All of the above.
E.  None of the above.

14.2    Classic Munchausen syndrome includes all of the following essential components *except*

A.  Travel from hospital to hospital.
B.  Simulation of disease.
C.  Unconscious self-induction of disease.
D.  Pseudologia fantastica.
E.  Use of aliases to disguise identity.

14.3    Patients with factitious disorder

A.  Often have a Cluster B personality disorder.
B.  Commonly have an Axis I disorder, especially schizophrenia.
C.  Have a need to be the center of attention.
D.  All of the above.
E.  A and C.

14.4    In studies of families with Munchausen syndrome by proxy, investigators have found all of the following commonly observed features except

A.  A dominant and aggressive husband and a caretaking and supportive wife.
B.  Intense family–group loyalty, with little protective concern for the child.
C.  A multigenerational pattern of abnormal illness behavior.
D.  Enmeshment of parent–child relationships.
E.  None of the above.

14.5    The form of malingering most frequently encountered by psychosomatic medicine specialists is

    A. Falsification of laboratory reports.
    B. Production of new illness.
    C. Contamination of laboratory samples.
    D. Embellishment of a previous or concurrent illness.
    E. None of the above.

# C H A P T E R   1 5

# Eating Disorders

*Select the single best response for each question.*

15.1   Eating disorders are among the most challenging psychiatric illnesses in practice and are associated with much psychiatric and medical comorbidity. Which of the following statements is *true*?

   A. Anorexia nervosa and bulimia nervosa are associated with a 5% mortality rate per decade of illness.
   B. Despite their lack of clinical eating disorders, semistarvation research subjects exhibited ritualistic behaviors similar to those of anorexia nervosa patients.
   C. Eating binges in bulimia nervosa feature foods composed primarily of carbohydrates.
   D. Most bulimia nervosa patients who seek treatment are overweight or obese.
   E. Progression from restricting anorexia nervosa to bulimia nervosa and normal-weight bulimia nervosa to anorexia nervosa are both quite common, about 50%.

15.2   Among the following illnesses in children, which is considered a feeding disorder rather than an eating disorder?

   A. Food avoidance emotional disorder.
   B. Pervasive refusal syndrome.
   C. Selective eating.
   D. Functional dysphagia.
   E. Pica.

15.3   Regarding the epidemiology and course of eating disorders, which of the following statements is *true*?

   A. Anorexia nervosa and bulimia nervosa are equally prevalent in young women, seen in about 1%–2%.
   B. Epidemiological evidence strongly supports significant recent increases in the prevalence of both anorexia nervosa and bulimia nervosa.
   C. Anorexia nervosa patients treated during adolescence have a more favorable long-term outcome than do those treated later in life.
   D. Among bulimia nervosa patients, less than 10% practice bingeing and purging 10 years after initial presentation.
   E. Anorexia nervosa patients with obsessive-compulsive personality traits have a better prognosis than do those with histrionic personality traits.

15.4   Laboratory tests that should be routinely performed in eating disorder patients include all of the following *except*

   A. Serum electrolytes.
   B. Blood urea nitrogen and creatinine.
   C. Thyroid function tests.
   D. Complete blood cell count.
   E. Serum amylase.

15.5 Psychopharmacological approaches to eating disorders may have an important adjunctive role in treatment. Which of the following statements is *false*?

A. For bulimia nervosa, all classes of antidepressants are effective.
B. Fluoxetine is the only U.S. Food and Drug Administration (FDA)–approved antidepressant for bulimia nervosa.
C. Medications alone have not been shown to produce long-term remission.
D. In general, patients with anorexia nervosa do not respond well to pharmacotherapy.
E. Olanzapine is a promising agent for treatment of anorexia nervosa solely because of its effect on appetite and weight gain, and it has been shown to be effective in controlled trials.


15.6 The most widely studied psychotherapy model for eating disorders is

A. Psychoanalysis.
B. Psychodynamic psychotherapy.
C. Cognitive-behavioral therapy (CBT).
D. Interpersonal psychotherapy.
E. Supportive psychotherapy.

# C H A P T E R   1 6

# Sleep Disorders

*Select the single best response for each question.*

16.1    Which of the following are polysomnographic characteristics of stage III/IV sleep in healthy individuals?

    A.  Spindles.
    B.  Slow eye movements.
    C.  K complexes.
    D.  Slow electroencephalogram (EEG) frequency.
    E.  A and C.

16.2    Regarding narcolepsy, which of the following statements is *true*?

    A.  In one U.S. community sample, narcolepsy was found to have a prevalence of 0.8%.
    B.  Narcolepsy is more common in women.
    C.  Narcolepsy is believed to be primarily a familial disease.
    D.  Narcolepsy commonly starts during the fourth decade of life.
    E.  Approximately 65% of patients with narcolepsy have cataplexy.

16.3    Symptoms of narcolepsy include

    A.  Excessive daytime sleepiness.
    B.  Sleep paralysis.
    C.  Episodic sleep attacks.
    D.  Cataplexy.
    E.  All of the above.

16.4    Essential signs and symptoms of obstructive sleep apnea are

    A.  Excessive daytime sleepiness.
    B.  Snoring.
    C.  Obstructed breathing during sleep.
    D.  A and C.
    E.  A, B, and C.

16.5    Regarding restless legs syndrome, which of the following statements is *false*?

    A.  The overall prevalence rate is estimated to be between 5% and 10%.
    B.  It is more common in older individuals.
    C.  Symptoms are worsened by activity.
    D.  It may occur in association with anemia.
    E.  It can develop during the third trimester of pregnancy.

# CHAPTER 17

# Sexual Disorders

*Select the single best response for each question.*

17.1 Sexual function in heart disease patients may be an important determinant of quality of life, thus affecting psychiatric status. All of the following statements are true *except*

   A. Sexual activity decreases and perception of sexual dysfunction increases after myocardial infarction (MI).
   B. Resumption of sexual intercourse with the usual partner and in the usual setting after MI does not affect cardiac morbidity.
   C. Decreased ejection fraction is associated with reduced libido and impaired sexual performance.
   D. Increasing exercise, losing weight, stopping smoking, and decreasing alcohol use all have been shown to reduce erectile dysfunction in cardiac patients.
   E. Sildenafil is safe and effective in stable angina if nitrates are avoided.

17.2 Sexual function may be adversely affected by several oncological interventions. Which of the following statements is *true*?

   A. Gynecological surgery for cancer typically results in a dramatic loss of sexual function.
   B. Decline in sexual function following prostate cancer treatment is attributable to erectile dysfunction, as libido and orgasmic function are usually unaffected.
   C. Sildenafil has been shown to be effective for erectile dysfunction after $^{125}$I seed implantation radiotherapy.
   D. In testicular cancer, sexual performance concerns far outweigh concerns about retrograde ejaculation and infertility.
   E. Intramuscular androgens are not effective in treating sexual dysfunction following bilateral orchiectomy for testicular cancer.

17.3 Sexual function may be a major concern for diabetic patients, and this area must be addressed in the context of other complications. All of the following statements are true *except*

   A. Erectile dysfunction in diabetic men correlates with increased levels of glycosylated hemoglobin.
   B. Depression in diabetes is associated with sexual dysfunction and other diabetic complications.
   C. Sexual dysfunction in diabetic men is typically limited to erectile dysfunction.
   D. Depression can produce abnormal nocturnal penile tumescence.
   E. The risk of erectile dysfunction is three times greater in diabetic patients than in the general population.

17.4 Renal failure, an illness commonly encountered in psychosomatic medicine practice, often affects sexual function. Which of the following statements is *true*?

A. Entry into long-term dialysis usually alleviates sexual dysfunction.
B. The prevalence of sexual dysfunction decreases following renal transplantation for both male and female patients.
C. In men, the impact of renal failure on sexual function is "central."
D. In women, the impact of renal failure on sexual function is "gonadal."
E. Erythropoietin in men with renal failure increases gonadotropic hormone levels but does not improve sexual function.

17.5 Psychotropic medications are commonly associated with decreased sexual function. This effect may be especially important in the medically ill. All of the following dosing strategies may be considered for selective serotonin reuptake inhibitor (SSRI)–induced sexual dysfunction *except*

A. Decreased dosage of the SSRI.
B. Change in timing of dose to several hours distant from anticipated sexual activity.
C. Drug holiday for clinically stable patient on a long-half-life SSRI.
D. Adjunctive bupropion.
E. Sildenafil.

17.6 The treatment of paraphilic disorders may involve the creative application of pharmacology. All of the following statements are true *except*

A. Pure antiandrogens (e.g., flutamide) are usually adequate monotherapy for paraphilias.
B. Medroxyprogesterone acetate (MPA) inhibits androgen biosynthesis and inhibits peripheral androgen action.
C. MPA has a "central" effect in decreasing paraphilic fantasy.
D. MPA is associated with weight gain, increased systolic blood pressure, and gallstones.
E. Leuprolide causes a transient increase in, followed by a profound suppression of, testosterone levels.

# CHAPTER 18

# Substance-Related Disorders

*Select the single best response for each question.*

18.1 Which of the following definitions or statements is *false?*

A. Physical dependence is a state of adaptation that manifests as a specific withdrawal syndrome.
B. Withdrawal syndromes are characterized by symptoms similar to those characteristic of use of the substance.
C. *Tolerance* is the need for increasing amounts of a substance to obtain the desired effect.
D. Addiction is characterized by craving and impaired control of drug use despite harm.
E. Psychological dependence is the feeling of need for a specific substance.

18.2 In Project Match, a large randomized trial of alcohol treatment modalities and predictive pretreatment variables, investigators found that the best potential predictor of a treatment outcome was

A. Social status of the patient.
B. Patient self-selection of treatment type.
C. Severity of addiction.
D. Number of previous treatment attempts.
E. None of the above.

18.3 Which of the following psychiatric disorders has *not* been reported to be associated with alcoholism?

A. Bipolar disorder.
B. Panic disorder.
C. Social phobia.
D. Major depressive disorder.
E. Schizophrenia.

18.4 All of the following are laboratory findings associated with alcohol abuse *except*

A. Increased serum gamma-glutamyltransferase (SGGT) level.
B. Decreased albumin level.
C. Decreased serum carbohydrate-deficient transferring level.
D. Increased uric acid level.
E. Increased mean corpuscular volume.

18.5   Buprenorphine is

    A.  A Schedule IV narcotic.
    B.  An opioid agonist at higher doses.
    C.  A short-acting opioid receptor antagonist.
    D.  A mu opioid receptor partial agonist.
    E.  None of the above.


18.6   All of the following are physical signs of phencyclidine (PCP) use *except*

    A.  Nystagmus.
    B.  Ataxia.
    C.  Pinpoint pupils at higher doses.
    D.  Hypertension.
    E.  Muscle rigidity.

# CHAPTER 19

# Heart Disease

*Select the single best response for each question.*

19.1 Depression and anxiety in heart disease patients may significantly affect quality of life and may complicate medical management. All of the following statements are true *except*

A. Depression is the most common comorbid psychiatric illness in coronary artery disease patients.
B. The prevalence of major depression following coronary artery bypass graft (CABG) is 20%–30%.
C. The prevalence of major depression in congestive heart failure (CHF) is 20%–30%.
D. Panic disorder occurs at a much higher rate in patients with mitral valve prolapse confirmed by echocardiography than in healthy control subjects.
E. Subsyndromal posttraumatic stress disorder (PTSD) is common in patients with automatic implantable cardioverter-defibrillators (AICDs).

19.2 A cardiac patient presents to a psychiatrist with a complaint of mood symptoms and of seeing yellow rings around objects in the visual field. The medication most likely responsible for these symptoms is

A. Reserpine.
B. Digoxin.
C. Clonidine.
D. Beta-blocker.
E. Alpha-blocker.

19.3 Regarding psychiatric aspects of cardiovascular disease risk, all of the following are true *except*

A. The mortality rate for depressed coronary artery disease patients is three to four times higher than that for nondepressed coronary patients.
B. Depression after CABG predicts an increased risk of recurrent cardiac events within the next year.
C. Depression is associated with worsened health status in patients with coronary artery disease, whereas decreased left ventricular ejection fraction is not.
D. In depression, heightened sympathetic activity and reduced vagal tone increase the propensity for arrhythmia.
E. The SADHART study demonstrated a statistically significant positive effect of decreased cardiovascular mortality with paroxetine.

19.4    Regarding cardiac transplantation surgery for end-stage cardiac disease and its psychiatric implications, all of the following are true *except*

A.  Patients awaiting transplantation commonly experience depression secondary to their helplessness to influence their own chances of survival.

B.  Patients on transplant waiting lists often experience guilt about the need for another patient to die to give them a heart.

C.  Patients on transplant waiting lists tend to minimize and/or deny their illness and to display ambivalence about the surgery.

D.  Patients awaiting transplant surgery are usually more anxious about the operation itself than about being excluded as a candidate.

E.  Steroid-induced mood disorder and other types of depression are seen in 20%–40% of patients during the first postoperative year.

19.5    Regarding cardiac implications of antidepressants and antipsychotics, all of the following are true *except*

A.  Tricyclic antidepressants (TCAs) can increase mortality in post–myocardial infarction (MI) patients with premature ventricular contractions (PVCs).

B.  Selective serotonin reuptake inhibitors (SSRIs) plus concurrent use of beta-blockers have been shown to lead to symptomatic bradycardia.

C.  Ziprasidone increases the QTc interval and has been associated with an increased risk of sudden death.

D.  A QTc interval greater than 500 msec contraindicates the use of haloperidol and thioridazine.

E.  Among the antipsychotics, thioridazine carries the highest risk of torsade de pointes.

19.6    Which of the following psychotropic medications is associated with a quinidine-like type IA antiarrhythmic effect?

A.  Carbamazepine.
B.  Valproate.
C.  Lithium carbonate.
D.  Lamotrigine.
E.  Buspirone.

# CHAPTER 20

# Lung Disease

*Select the single best response for each question.*

20.1 Which of the following statements concerning psychological factors in asthma is *false*?

  A. People with Cluster B personality disorders are more likely to have asthma.
  B. Brittle asthma patients are more likely to have anxiety disorders than are other asthma patients.
  C. Anxiety and depression are associated with more respiratory symptom complaints in asthma patients.
  D. Patients with asthma are more likely to hold catastrophic beliefs or cognitions.
  E. Asthma attacks may be provoked by psychological distress.

20.2 In patients with chronic obstructive pulmonary disease (COPD), anxiety and depression have been found to be associated with

  A. Higher relapse after emergency treatment.
  B. Increased disability.
  C. Lower exercise tolerance.
  D. Noncompliance with treatment.
  E. All of the above.

20.3 Regarding sarcoidosis, which of the following statements is *true*?

  A. Sarcoidosis affects white patients more than African American patients.
  B. In Europe, Italians have high prevalence rates.
  C. Onset of the illness usually occurs between the ages of 20 and 40 years.
  D. The disease follows a progressive, downhill course, with nearly 25% of patients dying from it.
  E. All of the above.

20.4 Absolute contraindications to lung transplantation include all of the following *except*

  A. Alcoholism.
  B. Anxiety disorders.
  C. Noncompliance with treatment.
  D. Hepatitis B virus.
  E. Cancer.

20.5 Theophylline has been found to reduce the effects or blood levels of which of the following psychotropic medications?

  A. Lithium.
  B. Fluvoxamine.
  C. Carbamazepine.
  D. A and C.
  E. A, B, and C.

# CHAPTER 21

# Gastrointestinal Disorders

*Select the single best response for each question.*

21.1 Peptic ulcer disease is a common gastrointestinal illness, with a substantial psychiatric component in many cases. All of the following statements are true *except*

A. The clinical use of nonsteroidal anti-inflammatory drugs (NSAIDs) has been associated with an increased risk of peptic ulcer disease.

B. The presence of gut infection with *Helicobacter pylori* is associated with the development of peptic ulcer disease.

C. The incidence of peptic ulcer disease has continued to increase since the 1960s.

D. A large-scale, population-based study (Goodwin and Stein 2002) found an increased risk of generalized anxiety disorder in peptic ulcer disease patients.

E. Psychological stress (as evidenced by anxiolytic use) is associated with peptic ulcer disease.

21.2 Inflammatory bowel disease (IBD), which includes Crohn's disease and ulcerative colitis, is commonly associated with behavioral and emotional factors, which may lead to involvement of the psychosomatic medicine physician. Which of the following statements is *true?*

A. Pathologically, ulcerative colitis is transmural, involving the full thickness of the gut.

B. Ocular involvement in ulcerative colitis is restricted to a retinitis.

C. The incidence of both Crohn's disease and ulcerative colitis has increased more than fivefold in the United States in the past 50 years.

D. Because of the seriousness of medical complications, IBD patients have a higher risk of comorbid psychiatric illness compared with irritable bowel syndrome (IBS) patients.

E. Among IBD patients, mood disorders are more common in older patients and in those with a history of previously diagnosed psychiatric illness.

21.3 Irritable bowel syndrome (IBS) and functional dyspepsia are considered to be functional gastrointestinal disorders. Which of the following statements is *true?*

A. The most common functional gastrointestinal disorder is functional dyspepsia.

B. The prevalence of anxiety and mood disorders in patients with functional gastrointestinal illness is between 30% and 40%.

C. Patients with chronic functional gastrointestinal disorders are more likely to present with anxiety, whereas first-time clinic patients usually present with depression.

D. Psychiatric treatment of anxiety and mood disorders in these patients is associated with improved health-related quality of life.

E. Patients with functional dyspepsia or IBS who consult physicians are less likely to have depression than equivalent patients who do not seek medical care.

21.4 Speech therapy has been found to be useful for symptomatic relief of which of the following functional gastrointestinal illnesses?

A. Globus.
B. Gastroesophageal reflux.
C. Functional abdominal pain.
D. Cyclic vomiting.
E. IBS.

21.5 Chronic hepatitis C virus (HCV) infection is a common gastrointestinal illness that often requires comprehensive multidisciplinary care. Which of the following statements is *not* true?

A. Chronic HCV infection is the major cause of chronic liver disease in the United States.
B. Major depression, posttraumatic stress disorder (PTSD), and other anxiety disorders are significantly more common in HCV patients than in control subjects.
C. HCV patients with end-stage liver disease (ESLD) have rates of depression similar to those of other ESLD patients (e.g., those with hepatitis B and alcohol-induced cirrhosis).
D. Depression is more common in HCV patients awaiting liver transplantation than in other patients awaiting transplantation.
E. Hepatitis B infection is less likely to be associated with depression than is HCV infection.

21.6 Antidepressant therapy may be helpful in managing IBS patients. Among the following classes, which has been clearly shown to be of benefit in IBS?

A. Tricyclic antidepressants (TCAs).
B. Monoamine oxidase inhibitors (MAOIs).
C. Selective serotonin reuptake inhibitors (SSRIs).
D. Selective norepinephrine reuptake inhibitors (SNRIs).
E. Trazodone and nefazodone.

# C H A P T E R   2 2

# Renal Disease

*Select the single best response for each question.*

22.1 Regarding end-stage renal disease (ESRD) in the United States, which of the following statements is *true*?

A. Each year nearly 80,000 Americans develop ESRD.
B. In 2001, more than 290,000 patients were receiving dialysis in the United States.
C. Nearly 8 million individuals are estimated to have chronic renal insufficiency.
D. A and C.
E. A, B, and C.

22.2 In a review of psychiatric illness involving 200,000 U.S. dialysis patients, it was reported that

A. Nearly 10% had been hospitalized with a psychiatric diagnosis.
B. Dementia was the most common psychiatric illness.
C. Compared with other medical illnesses, the primary diagnosis of depression was higher in patients with ischemic heart disease than in patients with renal failure.
D. A and C.
E. A, B, and C.

22.3 Dialysis encephalopathy, a serious cognitive disorder seen in dialysis patients in the 1970s and 1980s, was believed to be caused by

A. Azotemia.
B. Aluminum found in phosphate-binding gels.
C. Metabolic acidosis.
D. Hyperkalemia.
E. Hyperphosphatemia.

22.4 According to recently published U.S. guidelines (Moss et al. 2000), which of the following conditions is *not* an appropriate reason to withhold dialysis?

A. End-stage cancer.
B. Permanent unconsciousness (as in a persistent vegetative state).
C. Severe delirium.
D. Severe, continued, and unrelenting pain.
E. Multiple organ system failure in a hospitalized patient.

22.5 Which of the following forms of psychotherapy has been shown to be helpful in treating patients with end-stage renal disease?

A. Cognitive-behavioral therapy (CBT).
B. Hypnosis.
C. Behavioral interventions.
D. Group therapy.
E. All of the above.

# CHAPTER 23

# Endocrine and Metabolic Disorders

*Select the single best response for each question.*

23.1 The psychiatric care of diabetes mellitus (DM) poses several challenges for both psychiatric illness management and patients' global levels of health and functioning. Specifically, mood disorders are a significant problem in this population. All of the following are true *except*

A. Psychiatric disorders are associated with treatment noncompliance and vascular complications in type 1, but not type 2, diabetes.

B. The prevalence of depression in diabetic patients is two to three times higher than that in the general population.

C. Lustman et al. (2000) have postulated that depression and poor glycemic control are reciprocally linked.

D. Depression in diabetes mellitus typically antedates the development of vascular complications.

E. Conventional treatments for mood disorders in diabetes mellitus lead to improved glycemic control as well as improvement in depression symptoms.

23.2 Besides depressive disorders, other psychiatric illnesses are of clinical importance in diabetes. Which of the following statements is *true*?

A. The high risk of diabetes in bipolar disorder patients primarily relates to type 1 diabetes.

B. In bipolar disorder patients with type 2 diabetes, any excess weight is accounted for by weight gain from psychotropic medications.

C. The risk of type 2 diabetes in schizophrenia is approximately 1.5 times that in the general population.

D. It is believed that antagonism of $5\text{-HT}_{1A}$ receptors may lead to decreased levels of insulin and increased blood glucose in schizophrenic patients treated with atypical antipsychotics.

E. The increased risk of diabetes in schizophrenia is primarily due to the use of atypical antipsychotics.

23.3 Diabetes has been associated with effects on cognitive function. Which of the following statements is *not* true?

A. The onset of diabetes before age 6 years is associated with cognitive impairment.

B. In longitudinal studies of pediatric diabetes patients tested at 2 and 6 years after diagnosis (Northam et al. 1998), speed of information processing, vocabulary, and block design performance were worse in patients than in control subjects.

C. Recurrent episodes of hypoglycemia are associated with poorer learning and short-term memory performance.

D. Chronic hyperglycemia is associated with poorer visual organization skills.

E. The significantly increased risk for dementia in diabetes is due to the heightened risks both for Alzheimer's dementia and for vascular dementia.

23.4 Hyperthyroidism is a useful clinical model for psychiatric illness arising from metabolic disturbance. The symptoms of hyperthyroidism converge with those of several psychiatric illness groups. All of the following are true *except*

A. Presence and severity of psychiatric symptoms in Graves' disease correlate directly with thyroid hormone levels.

B. Graves' disease is associated with anxiety, depression, hypomania, and cognitive impairment.

C. According to Stern et al. (1996), the most common symptoms self-reported by hyperthyroidism patients were irritability, shakiness, and anxiety.

D. Anti-thyroid therapy is associated with improvement in depression symptoms.

E. Hyperthyroidism with anxious dysphoria is more common in younger, rather than older, patients.

23.5 Hypothyroidism offers another model of an endocrinologically based psychiatric illness. Regarding hypothyroidism and psychiatric illness, which of the following statements is *true*?

A. An elevated serum thyroid-stimulating hormone (TSH) concentration serves both to screen for and to confirm hypothyroidism.

B. Grade 1 hypothyroidism involves overt clinical symptoms, elevated TSH, and low serum thyroxine ($T_4$) concentrations.

C. Subclinical hypothyroidism is equally common in men and women.

D. Cognitive impairment in hypothyroidism may be independent of mood disturbance.

E. Subclinical hypothyroidism is most common in bipolar patients with euphoric mania without rapid mood cycling.

23.6 Adrenal cortical disease may readily come to the attention of the psychosomatic medicine physician. Notably, depression is commonly reported in Cushing's syndrome of excessive adrenocorticotropic hormone (ACTH). Which of the following depression-spectrum symptoms is *not* characteristic of a typical case of depression associated with Cushing's syndrome?

A. Hypersomnia.

B. Irritable mood.

C. Crying.

D. Decreased energy.

E. Suicidal ideation.

23.7 Various antipsychotic agents are associated with increased serum prolactin and resultant systemic complications. Which of the following atypical antipsychotic agents carries the highest risk of increased prolactin?

A. Clozapine.

B. Olanzapine.

C. Ziprasidone.

D. Risperidone.

E. Quetiapine.

# CHAPTER 24

# Oncology

*Select the single best response for each question.*

24.1 Many research groups have assessed depression in cancer patients. Cancer types highly associated with depression include all of the following *except*

   A. Breast cancer.
   B. Lymphoma.
   C. Lung cancer.
   D. Oropharyngeal cancer.
   E. Pancreatic cancer.

24.2 An increased risk of suicide in cancer patients is associated with all of the following *except*

   A. Advanced stage of disease.
   B. Inadequately controlled pain.
   C. Social isolation.
   D. Female gender.
   E. History of psychiatric illness.

24.3 Common causes of cancer-related fatigue include which of the following cancer treatments?

   A. Interferon.
   B. Chemotherapy.
   C. Irradiation.
   D. All of the above.
   E. None of the above.

24.4 In general, which of the following variables is associated with *less* mental distress in men with prostate cancer?

   A. More serious disease.
   B. Undergoing radiation treatment.
   C. Younger age.
   D. Undergoing surgery.
   E. None of the above.

24.5 One of the two most significant risk factors for breast cancer is family history. What is the other significant risk factor?

   A. Increasing age.
   B. Other physical illness.
   C. Autoimmune disorder.
   D. Depression.
   E. Past psychiatric illness.

# C H A P T E R   2 5

# Rheumatology

*Select the single best response for each question.*

25.1 Depression is a common problem in rheumatoid arthritis. However, consideration of the specific needs and complexity of these patients is important. Which is the recommended first-line pharmacological management strategy for depression in rheumatoid arthritis?

   A. Selective serotonin reuptake inhibitors (SSRIs), with doses limited to one-half the usual adult dose.
   B. SSRIs, in typical adult doses.
   C. Tricyclic antidepressants (TCAs), limited to low doses only.
   D. TCAs in low doses, routinely combined with SSRIs.
   E. Full-dose TCAs.

25.2 Regarding central nervous system (CNS) or psychiatric complications in rheumatoid arthritis, which of the following statements is *not* true?

   A. Neurological complications are common in rheumatoid arthritis due to direct CNS involvement.
   B. Psychiatric illness in rheumatoid arthritis usually relates to emotional reactions to having a serious systemic illness.
   C. Depressive symptoms correlate with levels of physical pain in rheumatoid arthritis.
   D. The association between rheumatoid arthritis and psychiatric symptoms is strongest for patients with more serious disease.
   E. Neuroticism in rheumatoid arthritis patients is associated with more distress, regardless of pain levels.

25.3 Which of the following is *not* associated with greater risk of depression in osteoarthritis?

   A. Older age.
   B. Lower level of education.
   C. Greater self-reported impact of osteoarthritis on patient's life.
   D. More pain.
   E. Objective measures of functional disability.

25.4 Systemic lupus erythematosus (SLE) is a complicated rheumatological disease known to be associated with psychiatric comorbidity. Regarding psychiatric manifestations of SLE, all of the following are true *except*

   A. Neuropsychiatric manifestations in SLE have a prevalence of between 75% and 90%.
   B. In SLE, the presence of antiribosomal P antibodies has been consistently associated with psychosis and severe depression.
   C. Antiphospholipid antibodies (e.g., anticardiolipin) are associated with stroke and cognitive impairment.
   D. SLE-associated psychosis, depression, mania, and anxiety are at least partially reversible with intervention.
   E. SLE-related cognitive impairment may respond to corticosteroid treatment.

25.5 Among the neuropsychiatric syndromes in SLE specified by the American College of Rheumatology (1999), which of the following is the most common?

 A. Mood disorders.
 B. Anxiety disorders.
 C. Psychosis.
 D. Cognitive dysfunction.
 E. Acute confusional state/delirium.

25.6 In the management of SLE, use of high-dose corticosteroids is necessary and thus common. Corticosteroids are themselves associated with psychiatric side effects. However, psychiatric comorbidity of SLE independent of the use of corticosteroids may make the sorting out of symptoms and causal factors difficult. Which of the following statements is *not* true?

 A. The reporting of severe psychiatric symptoms in SLE cases antedated the use of corticosteroids.
 B. Psychiatric symptoms are more common and more severe in SLE patients receiving corticosteroids than in patients being treated with corticosteroids for other illnesses.
 C. Psychiatric symptoms in SLE patients often improve with corticosteroid therapy.
 D. In SLE patients, reduction or discontinuation of corticosteroids may exacerbate psychiatric symptoms.
 E. SLE patients who experience psychosis during a course of corticosteroids usually will have a recurrence of psychosis with steroid retreatment.

25.7 Confusion, psychosis, mania, aggression, depression, nightmares, anxiety, aggression, and delirium have all been associated with which of the following medications for SLE?

 A. Gold salts.
 B. Penicillamine.
 C. Azathioprine.
 D. Leflunomide.
 E. Hydroxychloroquine.

# C H A P T E R   2 6

# Chronic Fatigue and Fibromyalgia Syndromes

*Select the single best response for each question.*

26.1   All of the following psychiatric disorders are among the exclusion criteria for chronic fatigue syndrome *except*

    A. Dementia.
    B. Anorexia or bulimia nervosa.
    C. Unipolar depression without melancholia.
    D. Alcohol or substance misuse.
    E. Bipolar depression.

26.2   The American College of Rheumatology (ACR) has developed diagnostic criteria for fibromyalgia. Which of the following are included in the criteria?

    A. Widespread pain.
    B. Symptom duration of at least 1 year.
    C. Pain at 11 or more of 18 specific sites on the body.
    D. A and C.
    E. A, B, and C.

26.3   Which of the following psychiatric disorders is most commonly found in patients with chronic fatigue syndrome or fibromyalgia syndrome?

    A. Depression.
    B. Psychosis.
    C. Anxiety.
    D. A and C.
    E. A, B, and C.

26.4   Which of the following is one of the best-supported biological abnormalities reported to be associated with both chronic fatigue syndrome and fibromyalgia syndrome?

    A. Low blood levels of cortisol.
    B. High blood levels of cortisol.
    C. Low cerebrospinal fluid (CSF) levels of substance P.
    D. Elevated blood pressure.
    E. Abnormalities of muscle metabolism.

26.5   All of the following medical disorders are commonly found in patients with either chronic fatigue syndrome or fibromyalgia syndrome *except*

   A.  Sleep apnea.
   B.  Rheumatoid arthritis.
   C.  Spinal stenosis.
   D.  Anemia.
   E.  Thyroid disorders.

# CHAPTER 27

# Infectious Diseases

*Select the single best response for each question.*

27.1 Pediatric autoimmune neuropsychiatric disorder associated with streptococcal infection (PANDAS) offers a compelling model for infectious disease–induced psychiatric illness. All of the following are true regarding PANDAS *except*

A. Seventy percent of children with Sydenham's chorea have obsessive-compulsive symptoms before the onset of chorea.
B. PANDAS consists of obsessive-compulsive and tic symptoms that occur following group A beta-hemolytic streptococcus (GABHS) infection.
C. The infection most commonly implicated is pharyngitis.
D. Antistreptolysin-O (ASO) titers rise with GABHS infections, and levels covary with symptoms.
E. Because of the high specificity of ASO titers in evaluation, throat cultures are superfluous.

27.2 Rocky Mountain spotted fever (RMSF) is another infectious disease that is associated with neuropsychiatric complications. Which of the following statements is *true*?

A. The responsible organism is *Rickettsia prowazekii*.
B. Central nervous system (CNS) involvement is seen in 25% of RMSF cases and includes lethargy, confusion, and delirium.
C. Irritability, personality changes, and apathy may occur before the rash in RMSF, most commonly in elderly individuals.
D. Encephalopathy in RMSF is rare unless computed tomography (CT) or magnetic resonance imaging (MRI) scans are abnormal.
E. Well over 50% of U.S. RMSF cases occur in the mountainous west.

27.3 Which of the following psychiatric symptoms is *not* characteristic of classic chronic Lyme disease encephalopathy?

A. Poor concentration.
B. Amnesia.
C. Fatigue.
D. Psychosis.
E. Depression.

27.4 Herpes simplex virus (HSV) infection can result in encephalitis that may come to the attention of the psychosomatic medicine psychiatrist. Which of the following statements is *not* true?

A. Electroencephalogram (EEG) testing is both sensitive and specific, with findings of periodic temporal spikes and slow waves.
B. Brain biopsy has a high diagnostic yield and a low complication rate.
C. Acyclovir is the drug treatment of choice.
D. Klüver-Bucy syndrome is a possible sequela.
E. HSV encephalitis is associated with olfactory hallucinations.

27.5    Viral hepatitis is a common clinical problem with psychiatric implications. Which of the following statements is *true*?

A.  Depression is a contraindication to interferon therapy.
B.  Fatigue in chronic hepatitis is more closely related to disease severity than to depression or social factors.
C.  Depression is uncommon in hepatitis C and B infections.
D.  Depression is induced in 20%–40% of patients treated with interferon.
E.  Depression induced by interferon is not responsive to selective serotonin reuptake inhibitors (SSRIs).


27.6    Meningoencephalitis with prominent somnolence, colloquially known as sleeping sickness, is associated with which of the following infections?

A.  Neurocysticercosis.
B.  Toxoplasmosis.
C.  Trypanosomiasis.
D.  Malaria.
E.  Schistosomiasis.


27.7    Which of the following antibiotics has been associated with psychosis, paranoia, mania, agitation, and a Tourette-like syndrome?

A.  Cephalosporins.
B.  Quinolones.
C.  Trimethoprim–sulfamethoxazole.
D.  Gentamicin.
E.  Clarithromycin.

# CHAPTER 28

# HIV/AIDS

*Select the single best response for each question.*

28.1 The most common neoplasm seen in AIDS patients is

A. Sarcoma.
B. Lung cancer.
C. Pancreatic cancer.
D. Colon cancer.
E. Lymphoma.

28.2 The addition of zidovudine to antiviral treatment regimens for HIV infection has resulted in

A. Worsening of cognitive functioning.
B. Improvement in cognitive functioning.
C. Onset of parkinsonian symptoms.
D. Increased risk for psychosis.
E. Increased delirium.

28.3 HIV is believed to increase the risk of developing major depression through which of the following mechanisms?

A. Chronic stress.
B. Worsening social isolation.
C. Demoralization.
D. Direct injury to subcortical brain areas.
E. All of the above.

28.4 AIDS mania often has a clinical profile different from that of primary mania. All of the following are characteristics of AIDS mania *except*

A. Irritable mood.
B. Infrequent spontaneous remissions.
C. Psychomotor agitation.
D. More chronic than episodic.
E. None of the above.

28.5 Which of the following personality characteristics best describes the majority of patients who would be seen in an AIDS clinic in a metropolitan area?

A. Unstable extrovert.
B. Stable extrovert.
C. Unstable introvert.
D. Stable introvert.
E. None of the above.

# CHAPTER 29

# Dermatology

*Select the single best response for each question.*

29.1 Atopic dermatitis is an often-chronic clinical problem with meaningful psychiatric comorbidity. Which of the following statements is *not* true?

  A. Emotional distress aggravates the symptom of pruritis in Alzheimer's disease patients with atopic dermatitis.
  B. Psychiatric comorbidity in atopic dermatitis is sufficiently common to warrant recommendation for routine psychiatric consultation.
  C. Various behavioral therapy models have been shown to reduce anxiety and depression in patients with atopic dermatitis.
  D. Topical doxepin cream has been shown to decrease itching in atopic dermatitis.
  E. Trimipramine has been shown to reduce nighttime scratching by increasing the time spent in stage I sleep.

29.2 Psoriasis is a chronic and relapsing dermatological disease of major importance to the psychiatrist, both because the disease is associated with significant psychiatric comorbidity and because it can occur as a side effect of psychiatric treatment. Which of the following statements is *true*?

  A. Lithium-induced psoriasis typically persists after lithium is discontinued.
  B. Bipolar patients who suffer from psoriasis due to lithium treatment should also avoid valproate, because of its similar risk for psoriasis.
  C. Psoriasis patients have been shown to be at high risk for comorbid personality disorders, including schizoid and avoidant personality disorders.
  D. Disability from psoriasis is more strongly correlated with disease severity and location than with psychosocial variables.
  E. Introduction of corticosteroids is correlated with triggering of psoriasis, but withdrawal of corticosteroids is not.

29.3 Delusional parasitosis is an unusual syndrome in which the patient believes that he or she is infested with living organisms. Which of the following is *not* true?

  A. Patients typically have experienced a specific precipitating event.
  B. Patients typically have had actual exposure to parasites.
  C. Patients usually readily accept psychiatric referral.
  D. Affected patients often respond to treatment with pimozide.
  E. QT prolongation from pimozide limits its use in patients with dysrhythmias.

29.4 Psychogenic excoriation may lead to substantial dermatological problems. Depressive and anxiety disorders are common in patients with this condition. Case reports and small open trials have shown some efficacy for psychotropic medications in psychogenic excoriation. Which two tricyclic antidepressants (TCAs) have been shown to be effective?

A. Nortriptyline and doxepin.
B. Doxepin and clomipramine.
C. Nortriptyline and desipramine.
D. Imipramine and doxepin.
E. Imipramine and desipramine.

29.5 Which of the following is *not* true of trichotillomania or its psychiatric comorbidity?

A. The mean age at onset of trichotillomania is after age 15 years.
B. Anxiety, mood, and substance use disorders are commonly comorbid with trichotillomania.
C. The comorbid personality disorders most frequently seen with trichotillomania are the Cluster B and Cluster C personality disorders.
D. First-degree relatives of affected patients have high rates of obsessive-compulsive disorder.
E. Clomipramine has been shown to be superior to desipramine for treatment, supporting an "obsessive-compulsive spectrum" construct for trichotillomania.

29.6 Lithium is notoriously associated with a range of dermatological side effects, which may limit its use. Lithium's dermatological side effects commonly include all of the following *except*

A. Skin pigmentation.
B. Urticaria.
C. Alopecia.
D. Psoriasis.
E. Exacerbation of acne.

# CHAPTER 30

# Surgery

*Select the single best response for each question.*

30.1 Which of the following are the elements of informed consent that a surgeon should include in his or her discussion with a patient about a proposed surgery?

A. Diagnosis.
B. Why the surgery is the treatment of choice.
C. Expected risks and benefits.
D. Alternatives and their consequences.
E. All of the above.

30.2 What percentage of children experience significant preoperative anxiety?

A. Less than 10%.
B. 10%–20%.
C. 40%–60%.
D. 80%–90%.
E. None of the above.

30.3 Risk factors for developing postoperative delirium include all of the following *except*

A. Older age.
B. Alcohol use.
C. Cognitive impairment.
D. Male gender.
E. Type of surgery.

30.4 Which psychiatric disorder has been found in burn patients during all phases (resuscitative, acute, and convalescent) of injury?

A. Delirium.
B. Posttraumatic stress disorder.
C. Alcohol abuse.
D. Mood disorder.
E. Cognitive disorder.

30.5 Bariatric surgery is usually performed for patients with extreme or morbid obesity. According to the National Heart, Lung, and Blood Institute guidelines, *extreme obesity* is a body mass index (BMI) of

A. $>15 \text{ kg/m}^2$.
B. $>20 \text{ kg/m}^2$.
C. $>25 \text{ kg/m}^2$.
D. $>30 \text{ kg/m}^2$.
E. $>40 \text{ kg/m}^2$.

# C H A P T E R   3 1

# Organ Transplantation

*Select the single best response for each question.*

31.1   Which of the following organ transplantations has the highest percentage of patient survival at 10 years posttransplant?

A. Lung.
B. Kidney.
C. Pancreas.
D. Heart.
E. Liver.

31.2   Psychosocial rating instruments may be of value in assessing patients' psychological preparation for and adaptation to transplant surgery. All of the following are true *except*

A. The Psychosocial Assessment of Candidates for Transplantation (PACT) provides both an overall score and a series of subscale scores.
B. The PACT can be quickly completed but requires scoring by a skilled and experienced clinician.
C. The Transplant Evaluation Rating Scale (TERS) rates 10 discrete areas of psychological functioning.
D. Because the TERS has more scored items than the PACT, it is more appealing as a research tool.
E. Between the two instruments, the TERS is considered to be more flexible than the PACT in terms of clinical use.

31.3   Factors that increase the risk of posttransplantation psychiatric illness include all of the following *except*

A. Pretransplant history of psychiatric illness.
B. Longer hospitalization.
C. Male gender.
D. Greater physical impairment.
E. Fewer social supports.

31.4   Psychiatric disorders may have an impact on the posttransplant health outcomes of patients. Which of the following statements is *true*?

A. Liver transplant candidates with Beck Depression Inventory (BDI) scores greater than 10 were more likely than nondepressed candidates to die while awaiting transplantation.
B. In liver disease patients with high BDI scores, the higher scores are attributable to a greater number of somatic symptoms.
C. In liver transplant candidates who receive transplantation, high pretransplant BDI scores predict poorer posttransplant survival.

D. In heart transplant patients, posttraumatic stress disorder (PTSD) related to the transplant surgery itself was not associated with a higher mortality rate.

E. Lung transplant patients without a presurgical psychiatric history were more likely to survive 1 year postsurgery compared with those with a psychiatric history.

31.5 Because of the complexity of posttransplant immunosuppressive and other ongoing medical therapy, treatment compliance is crucial to the ongoing well-being of these patients. Which of the following statements is *not* true?

A. Medical noncompliance in posttransplant patients is estimated at 20%–50%.

B. Noncompliance is a major risk factor for graft rejection and may account for 25% of deaths after the initial recovery period.

C. In the Dew study of compliance in heart transplant recipients (Dew et al. 1996), nonadherence to immunosuppressive medication regimens was the most frequent area of noncompliance.

D. Persisting psychiatric illness after transplantation is associated with medical noncompliance.

E. A "dose–response" relationship between number of risk factors present and rates of noncompliance predicts higher rates of noncompliance with more risk factors.

31.6 As is true in other areas of medical practice in which a high degree of personal investment in care is required for a successful sense of physician–patient collaboration, patients with personality disorders present special challenges for the multidisciplinary transplant team. Which of the following personality disorders is associated with the highest rate of posttransplant noncompliance?

A. Obsessive-compulsive.

B. Borderline.

C. Antisocial.

D. Narcissistic.

E. Avoidant.

31.7 Hepatic encephalopathy is a neuropsychiatric illness associated with end-stage liver disease that frequently comes to the attention of the psychosomatic medicine specialist. Which of the following is *not* true of hepatic encephalopathy?

A. Alteration of consciousness and cognitive impairment are common in hepatic encephalopathy.

B. Additional psychological tests (e.g., the Trail Making Test) may facilitate diagnosis in more subtle cases.

C. A major focus of treatment is to reduce the production and absorption of ammonia from the gastrointestinal tract.

D. Serum ammonia levels correlate well with degree of neuropsychiatric symptoms.

E. Anticholinergic medications should be stopped or avoided in hepatic encephalopathy.

# CHAPTER 32

# Neurology and Neurosurgery

*Select the single best response for each question.*

32.1    The classic clinical presentation of middle cerebral artery infarction in the dominant hemisphere includes all of the following *except*

    A.  Contralateral hemiparesis.
    B.  Neglect.
    C.  Aphasia.
    D.  Sensory loss of a cortical type.
    E.  None of the above.

32.2    Which of the following is a category or type of vascular dementia?

    A.  Subcortical ischemic dementia.
    B.  Multi-infarct dementia.
    C.  Dementia due to focal "strategic" infarction.
    D.  A and B.
    E.  A, B, and C.

32.3    Which of the following are core features of Parkinson's disease?

    A.  Tremor.
    B.  Rigidity.
    C.  Bradykinesia.
    D.  None of the above.
    E.  A, B, and C.

32.4    Pathologically, multiple sclerosis is characterized by all of the following *except*

    A.  Loss of oligodendrocytes.
    B.  Astroglial scarring.
    C.  Microhemorrhages.
    D.  Multifocal areas of demyelination.
    E.  Relative preservation of axons.

32.5    Which of the following statements concerning Huntington's disease is *true*?

    A.  Has a prevalence rate of 5–7 per 100,000 population.
    B.  Affects men more than women.
    C.  The most common age at onset is in young or middle adulthood.
    D.  A and C.
    E.  A, B, and C.

32.6  The brain region most commonly activated during partial seizures is the
   A.  Temporal lobe.
   B.  Parietal lobe.
   C.  Occipital lobe.
   D.  Frontal lobe.
   E.  None of the above.

# CHAPTER 33

# Obstetrics and Gynecology

*Select the single best response for each question.*

33.1 Infertility is a common clinical problem in obstetric/gynecological practice that is often fraught with psychosocial distress. Attention to and management of comorbid psychiatric illness may be an important part of infertility treatment. All of the following statements are true *except*

A. The prevalence of infertility has increased steadily since 1965.
B. Generalized anxiety disorder (GAD) is associated with lower rates of fecundity.
C. A higher trait anxiety level is associated with a lower pregnancy rate.
D. Comorbid depression is associated with lower pregnancy rates in women undergoing in vitro fertilization.
E. Infertility is associated with rates of depression similar to those in chronic illnesses (e.g., heart disease, cancer).

33.2 The pharmacological interactions between psychotropic medications and contraceptives may result in unwelcome clinical events. All of the following statements are true *except*

A. Implanted levonorgestrel metabolism can be enhanced by phenobarbital, decreasing contraceptive effectiveness.
B. Oral contraceptives inhibit the metabolism of tricyclic antidepressants, thus increasing serum levels.
C. Oral contraceptives enhance the metabolism of benzodiazepines, decreasing their effectiveness.
D. Modafinil increases the metabolism of oral contraceptives.
E. Carbamazepine and oxcarbazepine both enhance the metabolism of oral contraceptives.

33.3 Hysterectomy is a common gynecological procedure that frequently involves significant psychiatric factors. Which of the following statements is *true*?

A. Because it is associated with less surgical mortality, vaginal hysterectomy is now more common than abdominal hysterectomy.
B. Among women who undergo hysterectomy, African American women have the procedure at an older age than do other American women, on the average.
C. Women who undergo hysterectomy for chronic pelvic pain have better psychological outcomes than do women who undergo hysterectomy for bleeding.
D. Women undergoing surgical hysterectomy with oophorectomy are at risk for depression, especially if they have a history of depression associated with reproductive events.
E. Most studies show a decrease in sexuality in women following hysterectomy.

33.4 Chronic pelvic pain is an obstetric/gynecological condition associated with significant psychiatric comorbidity. Which of the following statements is *not* true?

A. Other somatic symptoms are common in chronic pelvic pain.
B. Patients with chronic pelvic pain frequently have a history of physical and/or sexual abuse.
C. The explanatory model of "psychogenic pain," wherein emotional pain is "displaced" onto the body, remains the most useful construct in understanding chronic pelvic pain.
D. Mood and anxiety disorders are common in patients with chronic pelvic pain.
E. Psychiatric diagnoses have been reported in 60% of these patients.


33.5 Psychiatric disorders that occur during pregnancy can be of great concern because of the challenges of managing a pregnant psychiatric patient. Which of the following statements is *true*?

A. Panic disorder patients who become pregnant should continue on medication throughout pregnancy.
B. Obsessive-compulsive disorder is likely to worsen postpartum but not prepartum.
C. Electroconvulsive therapy (ECT) for acute psychosis during pregnancy can be effective and is generally safe for the fetus.
D. Despite the later-appearing cognitive impairments, the perinatal mortality for fetal alcohol syndrome is less than 5%.
E. In "crack babies," the cognitive impairments are usually due to the toxic exposure to cocaine in utero rather than to social factors.


33.6 Postpartum depression and psychosis are among the most serious and potentially dangerous conditions in psychiatry because of their threat to infant safety. Which of the following statements is *true*?

A. Miscarriage increases the risk of depression in subsequent pregnancies, but stillbirth does not.
B. Postpartum depression incidence in North America is 30%–40% of pregnancies.
C. Thyroxine administration has been shown to decrease the risk of postpartum depression.
D. Antecedent anxiety disorder is a more important risk factor for postpartum depression than is antecedent depression.
E. Relatives of a patient with postpartum depression should typically offer to assume total care of the newborn.

# CHAPTER 34

# Pediatrics

*Select the single best response for each question.*

34.1 Which of the following is *not* one of Piaget's stages of cognitive development?

    A. Concrete operations.
    B. Informal operations.
    C. Sensorimotor operations.
    D. Preoperational thought.
    E. Formal operations.

34.2 Which of the following statements concerning failure to thrive (FTT) children is *incorrect*?

    A. Feeding problems and growth deficiencies can occur.
    B. Mothers of FTT children are reported to have experienced high rates of physical abuse.
    C. If a FTT child gains weight in the hospital, a psychosocial cause of the FTT should be presumed.
    D. Former FTT children have more behavioral problems than do children without a history of FTT.
    E. None of the above.

34.3 Which of the following statements about cystic fibrosis is *correct*?

    A. It occurs in approximately one of every 100,000 live Caucasian births.
    B. It affects approximately 250,000 children and adults in the United States.
    C. Less than 10% of patients with cystic fibrosis are adults.
    D. Eighty percent of patients with cystic fibrosis are diagnosed by age 3 years.
    E. None of the above.

34.4 Vocal cord dysfunction

    A. Commonly occurs comorbidly with asthma.
    B. Is often associated with anxiety.
    C. Can mimic asthma.
    D. Is associated with chronic stress.
    E. All of the above.

34.5 Which of the following statements concerning childhood obesity is *incorrect*?

    A. Children are considered obese if they have a body mass index (BMI) greater than or equal to the 95th percentile for age and gender.
    B. Recent data from the third Natural Health and Nutrition Examination Survey, conducted from 1988 to 1994, indicated that approximately 11% of U.S. children are obese.
    C. Increases in childhood obesity have not been documented in Asia.
    D. Children with a BMI at or above the 95th percentile for age and gender have significantly reduced health-related quality of life.
    E. Obese adolescents are less likely to complete college than are nonoverweight adolescents of similar educational backgrounds.

# CHAPTER 35

# Physical Medicine and Rehabilitation

*Select the single best response for each question.*

35.1 Which of the following is considered a less significant risk factor for psychiatric illness following traumatic brain injury (TBI)?

    A. Poor neuropsychological functioning.
    B. Preinjury psychiatric history.
    C. Preinjury social impairment.
    D. Increased age.
    E. Alcohol abuse.

35.2 Regarding post-TBI psychosis, which of the following statements is *true*?

    A. In TBI-associated psychosis, hallucinations are more commonly reported than are delusions.
    B. Right-hemisphere lesions are more common than left-sided lesions in TBI-associated psychosis.
    C. Seizure disorder rates in patients with post-TBI psychosis are higher than estimates for rates of post-TBI seizure disorders in general.
    D. The onset of psychotic symptoms is typically within 3 months of injury, with delayed onset after 1 year rarely reported.
    E. Negative symptoms are more common in post-TBI psychosis than are positive symptoms.

35.3 All of the following are considered risk factors for postconcussive syndrome *except*

    A. Older age.
    B. Previous TBI.
    C. Psychosocial stress.
    D. Male gender.
    E. Ongoing litigation.

35.4 Numerous psychotropic medications can be used to treat the symptoms of apathy and fatigue in central nervous system injury. Which of the following medications used for this purpose carries a risk of inducing seizures at usual doses?

    A. Modafinil.
    B. Methylphenidate.
    C. Dextroamphetamine.
    D. Bromocriptine.
    E. Amantadine.

35.5 Which anticonvulsant/mood stabilizer has been associated with paradoxical agitation in TBI and should thus be used with some caution and careful monitoring?

   A. Oxcarbazepine.
   B. Topiramate.
   C. Valproate.
   D. Lithium.
   E. Gabapentin.

35.6 The use of atypical antipsychotic agents in TBI may be helpful in controlling problematic psychotic and agitation symptoms. However, TBI patients are prone to delirium from anticholinergic drug effects and may also have an increased risk of seizures. For these reasons, which of the following antipsychotics should be used only with extreme caution in this population?

   A. Clozapine.
   B. Olanzapine.
   C. Risperidone.
   D. Quetiapine.
   E. Ziprasidone.

# C H A P T E R   3 6

# Pain

*Select the single best response for each question.*

36.1   The International Association for the Study of Pain (IASP) has defined *pain* as

A. An unpleasant, abnormal sensation that can be spontaneous or evoked.
B. An increased response to a stimulus that is normally painful.
C. An unpleasant sensory and emotional experience associated with actual or potential tissue damage.
D. An abnormal sensation, spontaneous or evoked, that is not unpleasant.
E. None of the above.

36.2   Visual prodromal symptoms, such as scintillating scotomata, are indicative of what type of headache?

A. Classic migraine.
B. Complicated migraine.
C. Constant (transformed) migraine.
D. Common migraine.
E. Hemicrania continua.

36.3   Which of the following statements concerning low back pain is *true*?

A. Nearly 25% percent of patients with acute low back pain will go on to develop chronic symptoms.
B. The least powerful predictor of chronicity is poor functional status 4 weeks after seeking treatment.
C. Economic and social rewards are not associated with higher levels of disability and depression in patients with chronic back pain.
D. Psychological factors highly correlated with low back pain include distress, depressed mood, and somatization.
E. The presence of an anxiety disorder has been demonstrated to increase the risk of developing chronic musculoskeletal pain 3 years later.

36.4   Using DSM-IV diagnostic criteria for somatoform pain disorder, researchers have estimated the lifetime prevalence of somatoform pain disorder to be

A. 5%.
B. 12%.
C. 17%.
D. 22%.
E. 34%.

36.5   During the first 5 years after the onset of chronic pain, patients are at increased risk of developing new substance use disorders and experiencing additional physical injuries. This risk is highest in patients with a history of

A. Substance abuse or dependence.
B. Childhood physical abuse.
C. Psychiatric comorbidity.
D. Childhood sexual abuse.
E. All of the above.


36.6   Regarding the use of antidepressants to treat pain, which of the following statements is *false*?

A. The selective serotonin reuptake inhibitors (SSRIs) produce weak antinociceptive effects in animal models of acute pain.
B. A study that used number-needed-to-treat (NNT) methodology to compare tricyclic antidepressants (TCAs) with SSRIs found that TCAs and SSRIs were equally effective in treating neuropathic pain.
C. In patients with chronic low back pain without depression, nortriptyline, but not paroxetine, significantly reduced pain intensity.
D. Drugs with noradrenergic activity are often associated with better analgesic effects than are agents with serotonergic activity alone.
E. Randomized, controlled clinical trials have not demonstrated consistent differences in efficacy among the TCAs.

# CHAPTER 37

# Psychopharmacology

*Select the single best response for each question.*

37.1 Protein binding may be affected by different disease states and may alter the concentrations of administered medications. Which of the following conditions is associated with an increase, rather than a decrease, in protein binding?

   A. Cirrhosis.
   B. Hypothyroidism.
   C. Bacterial pneumonia.
   D. Acute pancreatitis.
   E. Renal failure.

37.2 The serotonin syndrome is a potentially serious complication of serotonin-active medications. Its psychiatric presentation can include delirium, agitation, anxiety, irritability, euphoria, and restlessness, among other symptoms. Which of the following medications can contribute to the serotonin syndrome through its actions both as a serotonin agonist and as a serotonin reuptake inhibitor?

   A. Buspirone.
   B. Mirtazapine.
   C. Clomipramine.
   D. Tramadol.
   E. Nefazodone.

37.3 Anticonvulsants have an essential role in contemporary psychopharmacology but are associated with certain worrisome side effects. Among the following anticonvulsants, which is considered to be the most problematic in terms of cognitive side-effect risks?

   A. Topiramate.
   B. Gabapentin.
   C. Lamotrigine.
   D. Valproate.
   E. Carbamazepine.

37.4 The syndrome of inappropriate antidiuretic hormone (SIADH) results in a euvolemic hyponatremia. Several psychotropic medications are known to induce SIADH, and the psychosomatic medicine physician should monitor fluid and electrolyte status closely in patients taking these agents. Which of the following anticonvulsants has the greatest risk of inducing SIADH?

   A. Valproate.
   B. Gabapentin.
   C. Lamotrigine.
   D. Oxcarbazepine.
   E. Topiramate.

37.5 Clozapine is a revolutionary antipsychotic but has been associated with problematic and sometimes life-threatening medication side effects. Which of the following is *not* true of clozapine-associated cardiac side effects?

    A. Myocarditis, cardiomyopathy, and heart failure have all been reported.
    B. Most cases of myocarditis develop between 6 and 12 months after starting treatment.
    C. Myocarditis has been associated with eosinophilia.
    D. Cardiomyopathy has most often occurred in patients younger than 50 years.
    E. Clozapine withdrawal may improve cardiac disease.

37.6 Because of its potential for cardiac conduction problems, which atypical antipsychotic must be avoided in patients receiving drugs with quinidine-like antiarrhythmic properties?

    A. Clozapine.
    B. Quetiapine.
    C. Ziprasidone.
    D. Risperidone.
    E. Olanzapine.

37.7 Which of the following benzodiazepines is eliminated primarily by conjugation and renal excretion, and thus may be *less* problematic in liver disease patients?

    A. Alprazolam.
    B. Clonazepam.
    C. Diazepam.
    D. Oxazepam.
    E. Midazolam.

37.8 For the agitated patient without oral access, intravenous valproic acid may be a therapeutic option for the psychosomatic medicine physician. Which of the following is *not* true about intravenous valproate?

    A. Intravenous valproic acid (Depacon) was approved by the U.S. Food and Drug Administration (FDA) in 1997.
    B. The medication may be diluted in normal saline.
    C. The maximum infusion rate is 20 mg/minute.
    D. Cardiac monitoring is required.
    E. It is the only mood stabilizer available in parenteral form.

# Psychosocial Treatments

*Select the single best response for each question.*

38.1 Group therapy has shown considerable success as an adjunctive treatment for patients with a number of medical illnesses. Patients with which of the following disorders would be good candidates for group therapy?

   A. Heart disease.
   B. HIV.
   C. Breast cancer.
   D. A and C.
   E. A, B, and C.

38.2 All of the following are important tasks for group leaders in facilitating discussion among group members *except*

   A. Start and end the group on time.
   B. Follow the content and not the affect in the room.
   C. Respond to problems rather than accumulate unresolved difficulties.
   D. Bring group discussions into the room.
   E. Make each member feel that his or her problems are as important as anyone else's.

38.3 Hypnosis has been found to be effective in treating all of the following clinical situations or medical disorders *except*

   A. Acute procedural pain.
   B. Irritable bowel syndrome.
   C. Traumatic brain injury.
   D. Smoking control.
   E. Chronic pain.

38.4 Psychosocial interventions have been reported to benefit patients with which of the following medical conditions?

   A. Cancer.
   B. Heart disease.
   C. Diabetes.
   D. Arthritis.
   E. All of the above.

38.5  Which type of psychosocial intervention, as an adjunct to medical treatment for management of HIV, has most frequently been reported to be effective in reducing distress or psychiatric symptoms?

A. Cognitive-behavioral stress management (CBSM).
B. Hypnosis.
C. Interpersonal psychotherapy (ITP).
D. Brief psychodynamic psychotherapy.
E. Family therapy.

# C H A P T E R   3 9

# Electroconvulsive Therapy

*Select the single best response for each question.*

39.1   Although electroconvulsive therapy (ECT) is generally a well-tolerated procedure from a cardiovascular perspective, certain hemodynamic considerations apply. All of the following statements are true *except*

   A.  The barbiturate anesthetic used in ECT increases pulse rate and cardiac output immediately after induction.
   B.  After suprathreshold stimulation, the initial parasympathetic phase is followed by a sympathetic phase with tachycardia.
   C.  During the seizure, cardiac output increases by 80%.
   D.  Increased myocardial workload during ECT may be risky for patients with coronary artery disease and/or congestive heart failure.
   E.  Subthreshold electrical stimulation may lead to bradycardia and asystole.


39.2   Similarly to the hemodynamic effects of ECT, there are associated electrocardiogram (ECG) changes. Which of the following statements is *true*?

   A.  Sympathetically mediated dysrhythmic ECG changes in ECT include nodal rhythms.
   B.  Brief changes in the P-R and QTc intervals may be seen during and immediately following the ECT seizure.
   C.  Postseizure premature ventricular contractions (PVCs) are more intense if antimuscarinic premedication is used.
   D.  T-wave inversions in ECT generally herald myocardial compromise.
   E.  Increased T-wave amplitude during and after the seizure is seen in the majority of patients.


39.3   The depressed patient with chronic atrial fibrillation may benefit from ECT. However, certain precautions are necessary. Which of the following statements is *not* true?

   A.  Therapeutic anticoagulation should be maintained during the course of ECT.
   B.  In the patient not receiving chronic anticoagulation, short-term anticoagulation should not be initiated prior to ECT.
   C.  Transesophageal echocardiography to check for an atrial clot may be desirable.
   D.  The heart rate should be carefully controlled during ECT.
   E.  A beta-blocker as premedication may lessen ECT-associated sympathetic stimulation.

39.4   Parkinson's disease is a convenient clinical model for mood and cognitive disorders associated with a neurological illness. Because of the dual comorbidities of depression and dementia frequently encountered in these patients, the use of ECT is subject to some considerations specific for Parkinson's disease. Which of the following statements is *not* true?

A. ECT may improve the motor symptoms of Parkinson's disease.
B. Maintenance ECT treatment may extend clinical response.
C. Acute confusional states following ECT may be minimized by lowering the dose of Parkinson's medication.
D. Due to the severity of depression in these cases, thrice-weekly treatment is typically necessary, even in cognitively impaired patients.
E. Right unilateral or bifrontal electrode placement are preferred.

39.5   Regarding the use of ECT in depressed patients with comorbid epilepsy, which of the following statements is *true*?

A. With ECT, there is a progressive increase in the seizure threshold and increase in seizure length during a course of treatment.
B. Pre-ECT computed tomography (CT) or magnetic resonance imaging (MRI) of the head should be routinely obtained.
C. Pre-ECT repeated electroencephalogram (EEG) is generally required.
D. The patient's anticonvulsant regimen should be maintained.
E. Hyperventilation before the electrical stimulus may help to produce a seizure.

# CHAPTER 40

# Palliative Care

*Select the single best response for each question.*

40.1  Fully developed model palliative care programs ideally include all of the following components *except*

    A. Internet-based services.
    B. Intensive care unit.
    C. Home care program.
    D. Day care program.
    E. Bereavement program.

40.2  "Appropriate death" has been defined as

    A. Reducing internal conflicts, such as fears about loss of control, as much as possible.
    B. Sustaining an individual's personal sense of identity.
    C. Enhancing or maintaining critical relationships.
    D. Setting and attempting to reach meaningful goals, such as attending a graduation, etc.
    E. All of the above.

40.3  Regarding anxiety disorders in terminally ill patients, which of the following statements is *true*?

    A. The prevalence of anxiety disorders among terminally ill cancer patients and AIDS patients is low, in the range of 5%–10%.
    B. Prevalence studies of anxiety, primarily in cancer populations, report a higher prevalence of anxiety alone rather than mixed anxiety and depressive symptoms.
    C. Anxiety in terminally ill patients can occur as an adjustment disorder, a disease or treatment-related condition, or an exacerbation of a preexisting anxiety disorder.
    D. It is important to rapidly taper benzodiazepines and opioids during the terminal phase of illness to minimize the risk of dependence.
    E. None of the above.

40.4  Factors noted in patients with a desire for hastened death, in contrast to those without this desire, include all of the following *except*

    A. Depression.
    B. More pain.
    C. Pessimistic cognitive style.
    D. Personality disorder.
    E. Less social support.

40.5   Although words such as *grief, mourning,* and *bereavement* are commonly used interchangeably, which of the definitions below is the correct definition for bereavement?

A. State of loss resulting from death.
B. The process of adaptation, including the cultural and social rituals prescribed as accompaniments.
C. The emotional response associated with loss.
D. A pathological outcome involving psychological, social, or physical morbidity.
E. None of the above.

# CHAPTER 1

# Psychiatric Assessment and Consultation

*Select the single best response for each question.*

1.1 Clinical assessment of memory and executive functions is an important component in the diagnosis and management of cognitive disorders. Regarding clinical assessment of cognitive function, all of the following are true *except*

A. Having the patient register and then later recall specific information (e.g., three objects) is a test of working memory.

B. Semantic memory is assessed by questions of general knowledge and naming of common objects.

C. Declarative memory includes both semantic and procedural memory components.

D. Having the patient name as many objects in a category (e.g., names of animals) as he or she can within 1 minute assesses frontal lobe function.

E. The go/no-go test of ability to inhibit a response assesses frontal lobe inhibitory function.

**The correct response is option C.**

Declarative memory includes semantic and episodic memory components, both of which can be articulated, whereas procedural memory is implicit in learned action and cannot be described in words. Semantic memory is assessed by general-knowledge questions. Episodic memory is assessed by the patient's ability to recall aspects of his or her own history. Procedural memory deficits can be observed in patient behavior in interview. **(p. 6)**

1.2 Language disorders involve the dominant cortical hemisphere and are important in neuropsychiatric illness encountered in psychosomatic medicine practice. Which of the following is *not* true regarding clinical presentation and assessment of the aphasias?

A. Naming of objects is affected in Broca's (expressive) aphasia.

B. Naming of objects is affected in Wernicke's (receptive) aphasia.

C. Wernicke's aphasia overlaps with psychotic disorders in that both conditions feature poor insight and incoherent speech.

D. Conduction aphasia features impaired naming with preserved repetition.

E. Global dysphasia combines features of both Broca's and Wernicke's aphasias.

**The correct response is option D.**

Conduction aphasia features selective impairment of repetition. Global dysphasia combines features of Broca's and Wernicke's aphasias. **(p. 6)**

1.3    In the task of differentiating primary psychiatric from secondary medical etiologies of
       hallucinatory experiences, the affected sensory modality may guide the clinician to the more
       likely etiology. Which of the following types of hallucinations is often seen in substance abuse?

       A. Tactile.
       B. Auditory.
       C. Visual.
       D. Gustatory.
       E. Olfactory.

       **The correct response is option A.**

       Tactile hallucinations are often seen in substance abuse. Prominent visual, olfactory, gustatory, or
       tactile hallucinations suggest a secondary medical etiology, whereas olfactory and gustatory
       hallucination may be manifestations of seizures. **(p. 7)**


1.4    The adjunctive use of neuroimaging is an important part of psychosomatic medicine practice. The
       consultant often must determine which imaging modality is most appropriate for the clinical
       problem at hand. Which of the following pathological entities is better visualized by computed
       tomography (CT) than by magnetic resonance imaging (MRI)?

       A. Basal ganglia lesion (e.g., Parkinson's disease).
       B. Brain-stem lesion with motor signs.
       C. Cerebellar tumor.
       D. Acute intracranial hemorrhage.
       E. Vascular dementia with frontal lobe signs.

       **The correct response is option D.**

       CT is most useful in cases of suspected acute intracranial hemorrhage and when MRI is
       contraindicated, as in patients with metallic implants.
           MRI provides better resolution of lesions of the basal ganglia, amygdala, and other limbic
       structures and abnormalities of the brain stem and posterior fossa. **(p. 10)**


1.5    The electroencephalogram (EEG) may be a useful diagnostic tool in psychosomatic medicine, but
       it is subject to some important limitations. Which of the following clinical situations is most
       likely to be clarified by the use of an EEG?

       A. The search for a specific etiology of an established case of delirium.
       B. An insidious onset and slowly progressive dementia.
       C. Cognitive and motor deficits suggesting stroke.
       D. Distinguishing lingering delirium from schizophrenia in a psychotic patient.
       E. Localization of cerebral injury in traumatic brain injury.

       **The correct response is option D.**

       The EEG may provide concrete data to differentiate lingering delirium from schizophrenia. It
       may also facilitate the evaluation of rapidly progressive dementia or profound coma. However,
       the EEG is often not helpful in the evaluation of cerebral injury or head injury. **(pp. 10–11)**

1.6    Objective and validated standard test instruments have an adjunctive role in psychosomatic medicine, especially in the evaluation of suspected cognitive disorders. Which of the following statements is *true*?

A. Because of the ubiquity of cognitive disorders in psychosomatic medicine, the consultant should evaluate every patient with a standardized cognitive assessment.
B. The Folstein Mini-Mental State Examination (MMSE) is sensitive to subtle cognitive decline, even in premorbidly highly intelligent patients.
C. The Mini-Cog combines a clock drawing task with a concentration task (serial subtractions or reverse spelling) from the MMSE.
D. Clock drawing assesses temporoparietal and frontal cortical function.
E. Formal cognitive testing results are valid even if the sensorium is clouded.

**The correct response is option D.**

The Mini-Cog, unlike the MMSE, assesses temporoparietal and frontal cortical functions (via the Clock Drawing Test).

Standardized cognitive assessments are not needed for every patient. The MMSE is insensitive to subtle cognitive decline, especially in very intelligent patients. The Mini-Cog combines a portion of the MMSE (3-minute recall) with the Clock Drawing Test. Formal cognitive tests should be deferred until the sensorium clears. **(pp. 12–13)**

# C H A P T E R   2

# Neuropsychological and Psychological Evaluation

*Select the single best response for each question.*

2.1 All of the following statements are true about battery-based approaches to neuropsychological testing *except*

A. They are highly standardized.
B. They may require special equipment.
C. They generally are more time-consuming than patient-centered approaches.
D. They provide a comprehensive assessment of cognitive function.
E. They are very sensitive to neurological dysfunction.

**The correct response is option D.**

Battery-based approaches provide limited assessment of cognitive function, thus usually requiring the addition of other measures. **(pp. 16–17, Table 2–1)**

2.2 The Halstead-Reitan Neuropsychological Test Battery (HRNTB) consists of which of the following five types of measures?

A. Tests of verbal abilities.
B. Measures of spatial, sequential, and manipulatory abilities.
C. Tests of abstraction, reasoning, logical analysis, and concept formation.
D. All of the above.
E. None of the above.

**The correct response is option D.**

The HRNTB, the most frequently used neuropsychological battery in clinical practice, consists of five types of measures: 1) input measures; 2) tests of verbal abilities; 3) measures of spatial, sequential, and manipulatory abilities; 4) tests of abstraction, reasoning, logical analysis, and concept formation; and 5) output measures. **(pp. 16–17)**

2.3 Regarding the Minnesota Multiphasic Personality Inventory (MMPI), which of the following is *true*?

A. Many of the specific content scales are not sensitive to health concerns and neurological disorders.
B. An elevation in scores on scale 1 (Hypochondriasis) and scale 3 (Hysteria), with a significantly lower score on scale 2 (Depression), is referred to as the classic "conversion V" configuration.
C. Patients with seizure disorders, traumatic brain injury, or cardiovascular diseases have significantly lower scores on scale 1 (Hypochondriasis), scale 2 (Depression), and scale 3 (Hysteria).

D. Patients with rheumatoid arthritis often have elevated scores on scale 8 (Thought Disorder) and lower scores on scale 1 (Hypochondriasis) and scale 2 (Depression).

E. The presence of a conversion V proves the diagnosis of a somatoform disorder even without consideration of the patient's history, physical exam, or physical symptoms.

**The correct response is option B.**

Elevation in scores on scales 1 (Hypochondriasis) and 3 (Hysteria), with a significantly lower score on scale 2 (Depression), is referred to as the classic "conversion V" configuration. However, the presence of a conversion V does not in itself confirm the diagnosis of a somatoform disorder.

Many specific content scales of MMPI are sensitive to health concerns, neurological disorders, affective symptoms, thought disturbance, and ego strength. Patients with rheumatoid arthritis score higher on scales 1 (Hypochondriasis), 2 (Depression), and 3 (Hysteria). Patients with seizure disorders, traumatic brain injury (TBI), or cerebrovascular accident (CVA) score higher on scales 1 (Hypochondriasis), 2 (Depression), 3 (Hysteria), and 8 (Thought Disorder). **(pp. 23–24)**

2.4     Which of the following is an example of a projective personality measure?

A. Minnesota Multiphasic Personality Inventory (MMPI).
B. Millon Clinical Multiaxial Inventory (MCMI).
C. Thematic Apperception Test (TAT).
D. Personality Assessment Inventory (PAI).
E. Millon Behavioral Health Inventory (MBHI).

**The correct response is option C.**

Projective personality measures include the Thematic Apperception Test and the Rorschach inkblot test, which are designed to elicit responses that allow psychodiagnostic inference and detect disorders of reality testing and thought processes. **(p. 25)**

The MMPI, MCMI, PAI, and MBHI are examples of "objective" personality measures, in which the scoring of individual responses is based solely on an objective format in which all raters would agree. **(p. 22)**

2.5     Which of the following statements is *false*?

A. Objective personality measures provide qualitative information on personality structure.
B. Projective personality measures are time-consuming, sensitive to thought disorder, and provide rich psychodiagnostic information.
C. Self-rating symptom scales are standardized, reliable, and valid for psychiatric diagnosis.
D. Health-related quality-of-life scales are standardized, reliable, valid, and easily administered at bedside.
E. Objective personality measures and projective personality measures are time-consuming (45–60 minutes) to complete.

**The correct response is option A.**

Projective personality measures provide qualitative information on personality structure; objective personality measures provide quantitative indices of distress, coping, and personality style. **(p. 28, Table 2–3)**

# C H A P T E R  3

# Legal Issues

*Select the single best response for each question.*

3.1 The psychosomatic medicine specialist is often called upon to evaluate patients' ability to provide informed consent. All of the following are true regarding the doctrine of informed consent *except*

A. The *primary purpose* of the informed consent doctrine is to promote patient autonomy.
B. A *secondary purpose* of the informed consent doctrine is to facilitate rational decision making.
C. In emergency medical situations in which formal opportunity to provide consent is compromised, the law often "presumes" that consent is granted.
D. The determination of *emergency* is restricted to the patient's medical condition and not to availability of medical resources.
E. *Therapeutic privilege* is the exception to informed consent that is the least difficult to apply in practice.

**The correct response is option E.**

*Therapeutic privilege* is invoked when the psychiatrist determines that a complete disclosure of possible risks and alternatives might have a deleterious effect on the patient's health and welfare. Of the four possible exceptions to the requirement for obtaining informed consent, this exception is the most difficult to apply. Only rarely should it be necessary to invoke therapeutic privilege, because a skilled clinician should be able to explain the diagnosis and treatment in language that the patient can cognitively and emotionally accept. **(p. 39)**

3.2 Closely associated with clinical use of the informed consent doctrine is the determination of decisional capacity, in which the physician must render a decision regarding the patient's mental ability to appropriately participate in his or her own health care treatment. Which of the following is *true* of the psychiatrist's role in this clinical determination?

A. A psychiatrist at any level of training can declare a patient incompetent.
B. Only a board-certified psychiatrist can declare a patient incompetent.
C. Psychiatric illness is generally recognized by the law as rendering a patient incompetent even in the absence of cognitive impairment.
D. Adult patients are "presumed" competent unless they have been adjudicated incompetent or incapacitated by a medical illness.
E. The *Roe* case concluded that denial of illness was not grounds for a patient to be declared incompetent.

**The correct response is option D.**

An adult patient is considered legally competent unless he or she has been adjudicated incompetent or temporarily incapacitated because of a medical condition.

*Competency* refers to the minimal mental, cognitive, or behavioral abilities, traits, or capabilities that are required for a person to perform a particular legally recognized act. The determination of impaired competency requires a judicial decision; health care providers cannot declare an individual incompetent. Incompetence due to a psychiatric illness may not be recognized by the law unless the illness significantly diminishes the patient's cognitive capacity. The *Roe* case (*In the Guardianship of John Roe* [1992]) recognized that denial of illness can render a patient incompetent to make treatment decisions. **(p. 40)**

3.3    From their review of case law and scholarly literature, Appelbaum and colleagues (Appelbaum et al. 1987; Appelbaum and Grisso 1997) identified four key standards applied in the clinical determination of a patient's capacity to participate in health care decision making. Which of the following is *not* required to demonstrate decisional capacity?

A.  Ability to communicate a choice regarding treatment.
B.  Understanding of the treatment options available.
C.  Formal cognitive testing revealing an "unimpaired" range of performance.
D.  Appreciation of available diagnostic and therapeutic options.
E.  Demonstration of rational decision making.

**The correct response is option C.**

Formal cognitive testing is not required in order to demonstrate mental incapacity in decision making. In the order of levels of mental capacity required, the four standards for determining mental incapacity in decision making are 1) communication of choice, 2) understanding of information provided, 3) appreciation of options available, and 4) rational decision making. **(p. 41)**

3.4    General incompetence (as defined by the Uniform Guardianship and Protective Proceedings Act [UGPPA]) may encompass impairment from numerous causes. Which of the following is *not* considered grounds for a determination of incompetence according to this act?

A.  Minority status (age).
B.  Psychiatric illness.
C.  Advanced age.
D.  Drug intoxication or chronic use.
E.  Mental deficiency.

**The correct response is option A.**

Minority status is not considered when defining general incompetency under the UGPPA. **(p. 42)**

3.5    Regarding the *Cruzan* decision and its subsequent implications, which of the following statements is *true*?

A.  The court ruled that the state could not prohibit the removal of a feeding tube in a comatose patient.
B.  The state has an interest in the preservation of life, but not against the wishes of the parents of a comatose patient.
C.  Physicians must seek clear and competent instructions from patients regarding foreseeable treatment decisions.
D.  Decisions regarding future treatment require a durable power of attorney.
E.  All states have subsequently enacted legislation empowering surrogate decision makers.

**The correct response is option C.**

Physicians must seek clear and competent instructions from patients regarding foreseeable treatment decisions. This information is best provided in the form of a living will, health care proxy, or durable power of attorney; however, documentation by the physician in the patient's chart could serve the same purpose.

In *Cruzan v. Director, Missouri Department of Health* (1990), the court ruled that the state of Missouri could prohibit the removal of a feeding tube and that the state had an interest in maintaining the individual's life, even against the wishes of the family, because there existed no clear and convincing evidence of the patient's wish to have life-sustaining measures withheld under particular circumstances. Most states have consequently enacted legislation that allows surrogate decision makers to make critical end-of-life decisions in the absence of written evidence of the patient's wishes. **(p. 44)**

3.6    Advance directives are an increasingly important part of modern medical practice. All of the following are true *except*

A.  Health care organizations are required to inform patients of their right to advance directives.
B.  Health care organizations must inquire if patients have advance directives.
C.  A copy of the advance directive may be added to the official medical record.
D.  Federal law specifies the right to formulate an advance directive.
E.  All 50 states allow for the writing of a durable power of attorney for health care decisions.

**The correct response is option D.**

Federal law does not specify the right to formulate advance directives; therefore, state laws apply. Under the Patient Self-Determination Act (Omnibus Budget Reconciliation Act of 1990), all health care organizations must inform patients of their right to an advance directive and must inquire whether patients have made advance directives. All 50 states allow power of attorney agreements for health care decisions, and these documents should, if possible, be part of the official medical record. **(p. 45)**

3.7    The psychosomatic medicine physician may be called upon to evaluate a patient who has requested an "against medical advice" (AMA) discharge. All of the following are true regarding AMA discharge requests *except*

A.  The AMA form must be signed by the patient before the psychiatrist is called to evaluate.
B.  Failures in physician–patient communication are common in AMA discharge situations.
C.  External pressures (e.g., family responsibilities) often lead patients to request AMA discharge.
D.  Many AMA discharge–requesting patients have addictive disorders that have not been adequately diagnosed or treated in the hospital.
E.  The psychiatrist must evaluate danger to self or others as well as cognitive capacity for the AMA decision itself.

**The correct response is option A.**

There is no requirement that the AMA form be signed prior to the psychiatrist being called in to evaluate the patient. AMA decisions often occur as a result of failure in physician–patient communication, the existence of external pressure, or the presence of an undiagnosed addictive disorder. The psychiatrist must determine whether the patient is a danger to himself/herself or others and whether the patient possesses decisional capacity. **(pp. 48–49)**

# References

Appelbaum PS, Grisso T: Capacities of hospitalized, medically ill patients to consent to treatment. Psychosomatics 38:119–125, 1997

Appelbaum PS, Lidz CW, Meisel A: Informed Consent: Legal Theory and Clinical Practice. New York, Oxford University Press, 1987

Cruzan v Director, Missouri Department of Health, 110 S Ct 284 (1990)

In the Guardianship of John Roe, 411 MA 666 (1992)

Omnibus Budget Reconciliation Act of 1990, Pub. L. No. 101-508 (Nov. 5, 1990), sec. 4206, 4751 (42 USC, scattered sections)

Uniform Guardianship and Protective Proceedings Act (UGPPA), sec. 5-101

# C H A P T E R   4

# Ethical Issues

*Select the single best response for each question.*

4.1 The leading conception of the principles of biomedical ethics includes all of the following *except*

A. Respect for patient autonomy.
B. Beneficence.
C. Honesty.
D. Nonmaleficence.
E. Justice.

**The correct response is option C.**

The four principles that guide biomedical ethics are 1) respect for patient autonomy, which requires that professionals recognize the right of competent adults to make their own decisions about health care; 2) beneficence, to promote the health and well-being of the patient; 3) nonmaleficence, to avoid harming patients or research subjects; and 4) justice, which requires that medical care and research be performed in a fair and equitable way. **(pp. 56–57)**

4.2 You are called to provide a psychiatric consultation on a man hospitalized on the oncology service in a general hospital. The two key questions you should attempt to answer are

A. Does this patient have a medical or psychiatric disorder that compromises his capacity to understand, appreciate, and reason with respect to the details of a given diagnostic or therapeutic procedure?
B. Is this patient able to appreciate the differences between clinical care and clinical research with regard to the treatment options being recommended by the oncologist?
C. On the basis of your clinical assessment, should this patient be allowed to give or refuse permission for medical care?
D. A and B.
E. A and C.

**The correct response is option E.**

The psychiatrist providing consultation should provide first a clinical, then a moral judgment. First, does the patient have the capacity to understand the diagnosis and the treatment? And second, should this person be allowed to give or refuse permission for medical care? **(pp. 57–58)**

4.3 Which of the following sequences states the correct order of the continuum of decision-making capacity, from incapacitated to fully capacitated?

A. Able to assign a substitute decision maker → unable to make decisions → able to make medical decisions → able to appreciate the differences between clinical care and clinical research → fully capacitated.

B. Unable to make decisions → able to make medical decisions → able to assign a substitute decision maker → able to appreciate the difference between clinical care and clinical research → fully capacitated.

C. Unable to make decisions → able to assign a substitute decision maker → able to make medical decisions → able to appreciate the differences between clinical care and clinical research → fully capacitated.

D. Unable to make decisions → able to appreciate the differences between clinical care and clinical research → able to make medical decisions → able to assign a substitute decision maker → fully capacitated.

E. Able to assign a substitute decision maker → able to make medical decisions → unable to make decisions → able to appreciate the differences between clinical care and clinical research → fully capacitated.

**The correct response is option C.**

The correct order of the continuum of decision-making capacity is as follows: unable to make decisions → able to assign a substitute decision maker → able to make medical decisions → able to appreciate the differences between clinical care and clinical research → fully capacitated. **(p. 58, Figure 4–1)**


4.4 Regarding medical decision making, which of the following statements is *true*?

A. The parents of a disabled adult automatically remain the patient's legal guardians after their child's 18th birthday.

B. Studies have found that most (75%–80%) individuals fill out an advance directive for health care when given the opportunity to do so.

C. When an unmarried, incapacitated patient has an adult child, that adult child automatically is given medical decision making for the patient.

D. The completion of an advance directive for health care allows patients to specify in writing the medical care they wish to receive under various catastrophic medical conditions.

E. Substitute decision makers tend to base their decisions on what the patient would have wanted and not on what they themselves would have wanted had they been in the patient's place.

**The correct response is option D.**

The completion of a living will or advance directive for health care allows patients to specify their wishes about medical care under catastrophic circumstances.

The parents of a disabled adult do not automatically retain legal guardianship of their child after his or her 18th birthday, nor does an adult child automatically become the decision maker for an unmarried, incapacitated parent. Only 15%–20% of individuals fill out an advance directive for health care when given the opportunity to do so. Substitute decision makers tend to base their decisions on what they would want to have happen to them, rather than what the patient would have wanted. **(p. 60)**

4.5    Regarding the effect of major depression on medically ill patients, which of the following statements is *false*?

   A.  Major depression in medically ill patients often makes them decisionally incapacitated.
   B.  Untreated depression has been linked to poor compliance with medical care.
   C.  Depression produces more subtle distortions of decision making than does delirium or psychosis.
   D.  Refusal of life-saving treatment by a depressed patient cannot be assumed to constitute lack of capacity.
   E.  None of the above.

**The correct response is option A.**

Major depression in medically ill patients does not usually make them incapacitated.
   Untreated depression has been linked to poor medical compliance, increased pain and disability, and greater likelihood of considering euthanasia. Depression produces more subtle distortions of decision making than does delirium or psychosis, but refusal of life-saving treatment cannot be assumed to represent lack of capacity or suicidality. **(p. 61)**

# C H A P T E R 5

# Psychological Responses to Illness

*Select the single best response for each question.*

5.1 In "Personality Types in Medical Management," Kahana and Bibring (1964) cited seven personality types that overlap with DSM-IV-TR (American Psychiatric Association 2000) personality disorders. In regard to these personality types, which of the following statements is *true*?

   A. Dependent patients tend to adhere to treatment recommendations and have good frustration tolerance.
   B. Obsessional patients have high control and information needs and rarely exhibit conflicts between compliance and defiance.
   C. Histrionic patients should be required to directly confront their use of denial.
   D. Masochistic patients should be managed by reassurance rather than by acknowledgement of their chronic sense of suffering.
   E. Narcissistic patients' sense of entitlement should be reframed rather than being either directly reinforced or challenged.

**The correct response is option E.**

Physicians should not support the narcissistic patient's sense of entitlement, but rather should reframe it in such a way as to foster adherence to the treatment regimen.

   Dependent patients tend to adhere to treatment recommendations, but they have limited frustration tolerance. Obsessional patients want lots of information from their physicians but at times exert their need to control by refusing treatment or procedures. Histrionic patients should not be pushed to confront denial head-on. Rather than attempting to reassure masochistic patients, it is better to acknowledge their suffering and share their pessimism. **(pp. 71–75)**

5.2 The physician's countertransference response to patients is a crucial source of clinical data, both for understanding patients and for physician self-monitoring. Which of the following "personality type–countertransference response" pairings is *correct*?

   A. Dependent: feeling erotic attraction to patient.
   B. Obsessional: feeling little sense of connection to patient, finding it difficult to engage with patient.
   C. Histrionic: feeling powerful and/or needed.
   D. Masochistic: feeling angry, frustrated, helpless.
   E. Narcissistic: feeling overwhelmed, trying to avoid patient.

**The correct response is option D.**

Typical countertransference responses to a masochistic personality type include anger, hate, frustration, helplessness, and self-doubt.

The physician may feel powerful and needed when dealing with a dependent patient, or conversely may feel overwhelmed and annoyed, leading to a wish to avoid the patient. The physician may feel admiration for an obsessional patient or, in the extreme, may feel that he or she is in "a battle of wills," and may experience anger or an urge to counterattack. With a narcissistic patient, the physician may experience feelings of inferiority, or may enjoy a sense of status from working with an "important" patient. **(p. 72, Table 5–1)**

5.3 Folkman et al. (1986) identified eight categories of coping styles in a factor analysis of the Ways of Coping Questionnaire–Revised. A patient who acknowledges a personal role in a problematic situation exemplifies which of the following?

A. Confrontative coping.
B. Accepting responsibility.
C. Distancing.
D. Self-controlling.
E. Planful problem solving.

**The correct response is option B.**

The "accepting responsibility" coping style is characterized by an acknowledgment of one's personal role in a problematic situation. The other coping style categories are confrontative coping, distancing, self-controlling, seeking social support, escape-avoidance, planful problem-solving, and positive reappraisal. **(p. 76)**

5.4 Vaillant (1993) proposed a hierarchy of defense mechanisms ranked according to degree of adaptivity. Which of the following sequences (from a low to a high degree of adaptivity) is correct?

A. Psychotic, narcissistic, neurotic, mature.
B. Immature/borderline, neurotic, mature, adaptive.
C. Psychotic, immature/borderline, neurotic, mature.
D. Immature/borderline, narcissistic, neurotic, adaptive.
E. Immature/borderline, narcissistic, neurotic, mature.

**The correct response is option C.**

Mature defense mechanisms (e.g., altruism, humor) have the highest degree of adaptivity, followed by neurotic (e.g., repression, displacement, reaction formation), immature/borderline (e.g., splitting, idealization, devaluation), and finally psychotic defense mechanisms (e.g., psychotic denial, delusional projection, schizoid fantasy). **(p. 78)**

5.5 In Vaillant's (1993) hierarchy of defense mechanisms, a patient with a serious illness who consciously puts the illness "out of mind" is using which of the following defenses?

A. Suppression.
B. Repression.
C. Sublimation.
D. Displacement.
E. Intellectualization.

**The correct response is option A.**

This patient is using a mature defense, suppression, by consciously putting the illness out of mind. This response can be contrasted with repression, a neurotic defense wherein the person involuntarily forgets a painful feeling or experience. **(p. 79)**

5.6   *Denial* is an important and highly nuanced concept in illness and adaptation. Research has shown various effects of denial on physical outcomes. Which of the following statements is *true*?

   A. According to Hackett and Cassem (1974), myocardial infarction (MI) patients who were "minor deniers" had better clinical outcomes than "major deniers."
   B. According to Levenson et al. (1989), among angina patients, "low deniers" had better clinical outcomes than "high deniers."
   C. Among patients awaiting heart transplantation studied by Young et al. (1991), denial was associated with a worse survival rate.
   D. According to Levine et al. (1987), "major deniers" had shorter intensive care unit (ICU) stays but higher rates of noncompliance.
   E. According to Fricchione et al. (1992), increased denial was associated with more mood symptoms and sleep disturbance in renal disease patients.

**The correct response is option D.**

In Levine and colleagues' (1987) study, "major deniers" had shorter ICU stays and were more likely to be noncompliant following discharge.

MI patients who were "major deniers" had better clinical outcomes than did "minor deniers" (Hackett and Cassem 1974). "High deniers" among angina patients had better clinical outcomes than did "low deniers" (Levenson et al. 1989). Denial was associated with better survival rates in patients awaiting heart transplantation (Young et al. 1991), and greater denial was associated with decreased mood symptoms and sleep disturbance in renal disease patients (Fricchione et al. 1992). **(p. 81)**

5.7   Although anger is a common response to the threat of serious illness, anger in a patient often presents significant countertransference challenges for the physician. Significant anger under stress, such as when a clinical diagnosis remains unclear, is likely to be expressed by patients with all of the following personality disorders *except*

   A. Obsessive-compulsive.
   B. Paranoid.
   C. Narcissistic.
   D. Borderline.
   E. Antisocial.

**The correct response is option A.**

Obsessive-compulsive personality disorder patients are likely to become anxious (rather than angry), especially if the diagnosis remains unclear.

Patients with paranoid, narcissistic, borderline, or antisocial personality disorder are particularly likely to express anger in the face of medical illness. **(p. 82)**

# References

American Psychiatric Association: Diagnostic and Statistical Manual of Mental Disorders, 4th Edition, Text Revision. Washington, DC, American Psychiatric Association, 2000

Folkman S, Lazarus R, Dunkel-Schetter C, et al: The dynamics of a stressful encounter: cognitive appraisal, coping and encounter outcomes. J Pers Soc Psychol 50:992–1003, 1986

Fricchione GL, Howanitz E, Jandorf L, et al: Psychological adjustment to end-stage renal disease and the implications of denial. Psychosomatics 33:85–91, 1992

Hackett TP, Cassem NH: Development of a quantitative rating scale to assess denial. J Psychosom Res 18:93–100, 1974

Kahana RJ, Bibring G: Personality types in medical management, in Psychiatry and Medical Practice in a General Hospital. Edited by Zinberg NE. New York, International Universities Press, 1964, pp 108–123

Levenson JL, Mishra A, Hamer RM, et al: Denial and medical outcome in unstable angina. Psychosom Med 51:27–35, 1989

Levine J, Warrenberg S, Kerns R, et al: The role of denial in recovery from coronary heart disease. Psychosom Med 49:109–117, 1987

Vaillant GE: The Wisdom of the Ego. Cambridge, MA, Harvard University Press, 1993

Young LD, Schweiger J, Beitzinger J, et al: Denial in heart transplant candidates. Psychother Psychosom 55:141–144, 1991

# CHAPTER 6

# Delirium

*Select the single best response for each question.*

6.1 Regarding the altered affect frequently observed in patients with delirium, which of the following statements is *false*?

A. Increased irritability is common.
B. Affect is related to the mood preceding the delirium.
C. Lability is common.
D. Affect is usually incongruent with context.
E. Hypoactive delirium is often mislabeled as depression.

**The correct response is option B.**

Affect is unrelated to the mood preceding the delirium.

Anger or increased irritability is common in patients with delirium, and so is affective lability. Affect is usually incongruent with context. Hypoactive delirium is often mislabeled as depression. **(p. 92, Table 6–1)**

6.2 Regarding the epidemiology of delirium, which of the following statements is *true*?

A. The elderly are at higher risk of developing delirium than are younger adults.
B. Children and adolescents are at higher risk of developing delirium than are adults.
C. Up to 60% of nursing home patients older than 65 years may have delirium.
D. All of the above.
E. A and C.

**The correct response is option E.**

The elderly are at higher risk of developing delirium than are younger adults. Cross-sectional assessments estimate that up to 60% of nursing home patients older than 65 years may have delirium (Sandberg et al. 1998).

Delirium in children and adolescents has not been extensively studied. **(pp. 95–96)**

6.3 Which of the following symptoms, tests, or treatments can distinguish hyperactive from hypoactive delirium?

A. The electroencephalogram (EEG) shows diffuse slowing for hyperactive delirium and diffuse increased activity for hypoactive delirium.
B. Patients with hyperactive delirium are responsive to neuroleptics, whereas patients with hypoactive delirium are not.
C. Patients with hyperactive delirium have selective cognitive deficits, whereas patients with hypoactive delirium have diffuse cognitive deficits.
D. Patients with hyperactive delirium have higher mortality rates, whereas patients with hypoactive delirium have lower mortality rates.

E.  Delirium due to drug-related causes is most commonly hyperactive, whereas delirium due to metabolic disturbances is more frequently hypoactive.

**The correct response is option E.**

Delirium due to drug-related causes is most commonly hyperactive, whereas delirium due to metabolic disturbances, including hypoxia, is more frequently hypoactive.

The EEG shows diffuse slowing for both hypo- and hyperactive delirium. Patients with hyperactive delirium and with hypoactive delirium are equally responsive to neuroleptics. Diffuse cognitive deficits are present in both hyperactive delirium and hypoactive delirium. Patients with hyperactive delirium have lower mortality rates than do patients with hypoactive delirium. **(p. 106, Table 6–4)**

6.4  Regarding delirium assessment instruments, which of the following statements is *true*?

A.  The Confusion Assessment Method (CAM) is based on DSM-III-R (American Psychiatric Association 1987) criteria and is intended for use by nonpsychiatric clinicians in a hospital setting.
B.  The Delirium Rating Scale (DRS) has two forms—a full-scale 11-item form and a 4-item form.
C.  The Memorial Delirium Assessment Scale (MDAS) is a 10-item scale assessing a breadth of delirium features and can function both to clarify diagnosis and to assess symptom severity because of its hierarchical nature.
D.  The delirium assessment tool most commonly used by nurses is the Delirium Rating Scale—Revised–98 (DRS-R-98), a 30-point scale with cutoffs for levels of confusion severity.
E.  The Organic Brain Syndrome Scale is based on DSM-IV (American Psychiatric Association 1994) criteria and includes 16 items, with 3 diagnostic items separable from 13 severity items that form a severity scale.

**The correct response is option A.**

The CAM, the most widely used screening tool for diagnosis of delirium in general hospitals, is based on DSM-III-R criteria, is intended for use by nonpsychiatric clinicians, and is useful for case finding.

The DRS is a 10-item scale that can function both to clarify diagnosis and to assess symptom severity. The MDAS is a 10-item, severity-rating scale for use after a diagnosis of delirium has been made. The NEECHAM Scale is the delirium assessment tool most commonly used by nurses. The DRS-R-98 has 16 items, with 3 diagnostic items separable from 13 severity items that form a severity subscale. The Organic Brain Syndrome Scale is based on DSM-III (American Psychiatric Association 1980)–derived items rated along a continuum of mild to moderate to severe. **(pp. 108–109)**

6.5  The EEG finding most typically seen in patients with delirium is

A.  Low-voltage fast activity.
B.  Diffuse slowing.
C.  Frontocentral spikes.
D.  Delta bursts.
E.  None of the above.

**The correct response is option B.**

Diffuse slowing is the most typical EEG pattern found in delirium.

Low-voltage fast activity is typical of delirium tremens. Frontocentral spikes are caused by hypnosedative drug withdrawal or by tricyclic antidepressant and phenothiazine intoxication. Delta burst are most often seen in adolescents with acute confusional migraine. **(p. 111)**

6.6    The best-established neurotransmitter alteration in delirium is

    A. Increased dopaminergic activity.
    B. Increased cholinergic activity.
    C. Increased gamma-aminobutyric acid (GABA)ergic activity.
    D. Decreased serotonergic activity.
    E. Decreased cholinergic activity.

**The correct response is option E.**

The best-established neurotransmitter alteration, accounting for many cases of delirium, is reduced cholinergic activity (Trzepacz 1996, 2000). **(pp. 113–114)**

# References

American Psychiatric Association: Diagnostic and Statistical Manual of Mental Disorders, 3rd Edition. Washington, DC, American Psychiatric Association, 1980

American Psychiatric Association: Diagnostic and Statistical Manual of Mental Disorders, 3rd Edition, Revised. Washington, DC, American Psychiatric Association, 1987

American Psychiatric Association: Diagnostic and Statistical Manual of Mental Disorders, 4th Edition. Washington, DC, American Psychiatric Association, 1994

Sandberg O, Gustafson Y, Brannstrom B, et al: Prevalence of dementia, delirium and psychiatric symptoms in various care settings for the elderly. Scand J Soc Med 26:56–62, 1998

Trzepacz PT: Anticholinergic model for delirium. Semin Clin Neuropsychiatry 1:294–303, 1996

Trzepacz PT: Is there a final common neural pathway in delirium? focus on acetylcholine and dopamine. Semin Clin Neuropsychiatry 5:132–148, 2000

# C H A P T E R   7

# Dementia

*Select the single best response for each question.*

7.1    The distinction of cortical versus subcortical dementia provides a clinically useful framework for classification of clinical symptoms and dementia syndromes. Among the following neurodegenerative disorders that lead to dementia, which one most typically results in cortical dementia?

A.  Dementia with Lewy bodies.
B.  Parkinson's disease.
C.  Huntington's disease.
D.  Wilson's disease.
E.  Progressive supranuclear palsy.

**The correct response is option A.**

Dementia with Lewy bodies most typically results in cortical dementia. Parkinson's disease, Huntington's disease, Wilson's disease, and progressive supranuclear palsy result in subcortical dementia. **(p. 133)**

7.2    In dementia of the Alzheimer's type (DAT), numerous putatively protective factors have been proposed. Which of the following proposed protective factors is considered confirmed?

A.  Low cholesterol.
B.  Apolipoprotein ε3 allele.
C.  Apolipoprotein ε2 allele.
D.  Statin drugs.
E.  Vitamin E.

**The correct response is option C.**

The apolipoprotein ε2 allele is considered a confirmed protective factor for DAT and is also considered a protective factor for vascular dementia. Whether low cholesterol level, statin drugs, and vitamin E are protective against DAT is controversial. **(p. 135, Table 7–4)**

7.3    In vascular dementia, numerous risk factors have been identified that roughly parallel the risk for coronary artery disease. Which of the following vascular dementia risk factors is considered confirmed?

A.  Atrial fibrillation.
B.  Hypertension.
C.  Excess alcohol use.
D.  Hyperlipidemia.
E.  Female sex.

**The correct response is option B.**

Hypertension, in addition to cigarette smoking and diabetes mellitus, has been shown to be a risk factor for vascular dementia. **(p. 135, Table 7–4)**

7.4   Cortical dementia (of which dementia of the Alzheimer's type is the prototype) can be identified by a common constellation of specific cognitive symptoms. All of the following symptoms are consistent with cortical dementia *except*

  A. Apathy leading to akinetic mutism.
  B. Amnesia which is not helped by cueing.
  C. Aphasia.
  D. Apraxia.
  E. Agnosia.

**The correct response is option A.**

Amnesia, aphasia, apraxia, and agnosia are all symptoms of cortical dementia. Apathy that leads to akinetic mutism is a sign of subcortical dementia. **(p. 138)**

7.5   The distinction of cortical versus subcortical dementia on clinical grounds may be an important differentiation in clinical practice. Which of the following clinical findings is more consistent with subcortical than with cortical dementia?

  A. Normal gait.
  B. Loss of initiative.
  C. Less frequent mood symptoms.
  D. Pathological reflexes.
  E. Absence of extrapyramidal side effects (EPS).

**The correct response is option B.**

Loss of initiative is a marked sign of subcortical dementia, which is characterized by the predominant involvement of the white matter and deep gray matter structures (basal ganglia, thalamus, frontal lobe projections). **(p. 139, Table 7–6)**

7.6   In frontotemporal dementia, all of the following symptoms or signs are typical *except*

  A. Irritability.
  B. Decreases in social judgment.
  C. Decreased impulse control with acting out.
  D. Early cognitive impairment.
  E. Hyperorality.

**The correct response is option D.**

In frontotemporal dementia, personality changes and neuropsychiatric symptoms precede cognitive decline by several years. Psychiatric symptoms include irritability; poor judgment; decreased impulse control, including acting out; disinhibition; and a general disregard for the conventional rules of social conduct. **(p. 140)**

7.7    Prognosis in dementia of the Alzheimer's type is an important aspect of clinical care for these patients. Which of the following statements is *true*?

A.  Progression of deterioration is usually 4–6 Mini-Mental State Examination (MMSE) points per year.
B.  Cognitive deterioration is more rapid if Lewy bodies are absent.
C.  Psychotic symptoms at baseline portend more rapid decline.
D.  Delusions and/or hallucinations are more persistent than agitation and depression as the disease progresses.
E.  Basic activities of daily living (ADLs) are more seriously impaired than are instrumental ADLs.

**The correct response is option C.**

Psychotic symptoms at baseline strongly and independently portend a more rapid decline in dementia of the Alzheimer's type. **(p. 152)**

   Progression of deterioration is usually 2–4 MMSE points per year. Cognitive deterioration is more rapid if Lewy bodies are present. As the disease progresses, depression, agitation, and aggression are more persistent than delusions and hallucination. Instrumental ADLs are impaired earlier than are basic ADLs. **(p. 140)**


7.8    Among the following medications, which antipsychotic agent would be preferred in Parkinson's disease or Lewy body dementia presenting with psychosis and agitation?

A.  Haloperidol.
B.  Chlorpromazine.
C.  Risperidone.
D.  Clozapine.
E.  Thioridazine.

**The correct response is option D.**

Among the medications listed, clozapine is the best choice for Parkinson's disease or dementia with Lewy bodies.

   Haloperidol, risperidone, olanzapine, quetiapine, and ziprasidone are also used in dementia, but thioridazine, which has high anticholinergic activity, may cause worrisome QT prolongation. **(p. 153)**

# CHAPTER 8

# Aggression and Violence

*Select the single best response for each question.*

8.1    Which of the following characteristics are usually *not* indicative of impulsive aggression?

    A.  Unplanned.
    B.  Explosive.
    C.  Deliberate.
    D.  All of the above.
    E.  None of the above.

**The correct response is option C.**

Impulsive aggression is relatively unplanned and sometimes explosive, whereas premeditated aggression is deliberate behavior that may be predatory. **(p. 174)**

8.2    Which of the following statements concerning aggression is *true*?

    A.  Aggression and violence in inpatient settings appear to be relatively frequent in the 24 hours immediately prior to discharge.
    B.  Involuntary admission rarely precipitates aggressive acts and violence.
    C.  Substance users may become aggressive soon after admission.
    D.  A rapid increase in the risk of aggression in patients with schizophrenia within a few days after admission is common.
    E.  Patient–staff conflicts, such as the denial of privileges, rarely precipitates aggression.

**The correct response is option C.**

Substance users may become aggressive soon after admission as a result of irritability associated with withdrawal.

    Aggression and violence in inpatient settings appear to be relatively frequent in the 48 hours after admission. A rapid reduction in the risk of aggression is seen in patients with schizophrenia within a few days after admission. Patient–staff conflicts can precipitate aggressive acts and violence, especially in situations involving enforcement of rules or denial of privileges. **(p. 175)**

8.3    The neurotransmitter system(s) involved in the modulation of aggression include

    A.  Serotonin.
    B.  Norepinephrine.
    C.  Dopamine.
    D.  All of the above.
    E.  None of the above.

**The correct response is option D.**

The neurotransmitter systems responsible for the modulation of aggression are primarily those involving serotonin and the catecholamines (norepinephrine and dopamine). **(p. 176)**

8.4   The diagnostic term *intermittent explosive disorder*

    A. Refers to recurrent episodes of explosive anger not explained by psychosis or some other mental disorder.

    B. Has been used to describe rage attacks in association with lesions of the hypothalamus and amygdala.

    C. Has been used as a label for males with a history of conduct disorder.

    D. May be applied to individuals with antisocial personality disorder who exhibit uncontrollable rage.

    E. Can be used as an additional diagnosis for individuals with attention-deficit/hyperactivity disorder (ADHD) who show symptoms of explosive anger.

**The correct response is option A.**

*Intermittent explosive disorder* refers to a disturbance characterized by recurrent episodes of explosive anger not explained by psychosis or some other mental disorder.

    *Episodic dyscontrol syndrome*, denoting recurring episodes of uncontrollable rage, has been used as a label for males with a history of conduct disorder, unstable employment, poverty, domestic violence and other sexual assaults, criminal behavior, and substance abuse. Episodic dyscontrol syndrome overlaps with ADHD, conduct disorder, and antisocial personality disorder. Rage attacks in association with lesions of the hypothalamus and amygdala are termed *hypothalamic rage attacks* or *hypothalamic-limbic rage syndrome.* **(p. 180)**

8.5   Effective de-escalation techniques for controlling and terminating mild to moderate aggression in hospital settings include all of the following *except*

    A. Maintain a safe distance.

    B. Avoid sudden movements.

    C. Avoid personalizing yourself.

    D. Stay at the same height as the patient.

    E. Do not touch the patient.

**The correct response is option C.**

Personalizing oneself is an effective verbal de-escalation technique for the clinician.

    Maintaining a safe distance, avoiding sudden movements, staying at the same height as the patient, not touching the patient, maintaining a neutral posture, and refraining from staring are effective nonverbal techniques. **(p. 185)**

# CHAPTER 9

# Depression

*Select the single best response for each question.*

9.1 Depression rating scales may be helpful to the clinician in detecting mood symptoms in medically ill patients. Which of the following statements is *true*?

A. The Center for Epidemiologic Studies Depression Scale (CES-D) is a 20-item scale validated for use in the medically ill.
B. The Hospital Anxiety and Depression Scale (HADS) is useful in medically ill populations because it assesses many somatic symptoms of depression.
C. The Beck Depression Inventory–II (BDI-II) is only moderately valid in medically ill patients, because it addresses few somatic symptoms.
D. The Patient Health Questionnaire (PHQ) requires clinician administration.
E. The HADS has better sensitivity and specificity for depression in medical illness than does the PHQ.

**The correct response is option A.**

The CES-D scale is a 20-item self-report measure of depressive symptoms that has been extensively used in medically ill samples, with evidence of good psychometric properties.

The HADS is a 14-item self-report scale with separate 7-item subscales for anxiety and depression. The depression subscale does not include somatic items. The BDI-II can be used effectively to screen for depression in the medically ill. The PHQ is a self-administered version of the PRIME-MD. The PHQ has better sensitivity and specificity than does the HADS. **(pp. 198–199)**

9.2 The interrelationship between coronary artery disease (CAD) and depression is complex but clinically important to psychosomatic medicine practice. All of the following are true *except*

A. Depression increases morbidity and mortality risk in CAD.
B. The American College of Cardiology regards depression as a primary risk factor for CAD.
C. CAD patients with depression have an increased neuroendocrine response to stress.
D. The Sertraline Antidepressant Heart Attack Trial (SADHART) found only modest effects of sertraline on cardiac function.
E. The Enhancing Recovery in Coronary Heart Disease (ENRICHD) study, which used cognitive-behavioral therapy (CBT) and selective serotonin reuptake inhibitors (SSRIs), found no decrease in recurrent myocardial infarction (MI) risk with these interventions.

**The correct response is option B.**

The American College of Cardiology regards depression as a secondary risk factor for CAD.

Depressed mood is an independent predictor of morbidity and mortality following the onset of CAD. CAD patients have increased sympathetic and neuroendocrine response to stress. The SADHART failed to demonstrate improvement of cardiovascular functioning (Glassman et al. 2002), whereas the ENRICHD trial failed to show a decrease in recurrent MI risk or mortality (Berkman et al. 2003). **(pp. 200–201)**

9.3    The relationship between depression and cancer is also important in psychosomatic medicine. Many specific cancer sites are associated with a notably higher risk for depression. Which of the following is *not* generally associated with a significantly higher risk for depression?

A.  Lung cancer.
B.  Pancreatic cancer.
C.  Central nervous system (CNS) cancer.
D.  Oropharyngeal cancer.
E.  Skin cancer.

**The correct response is option E.**

Prevalence rates for depression in cancer are between 10% and 30%. Higher rates of depression are associated with certain cancer types, such as lung, pancreas, brain, and oropharynx tumors. Skin cancer is not generally associated with a significant risk for depression. **(p. 201)**

9.4    Depression and neurological disease are commonly comorbid. All of the following statements are true regarding depression in neurological disease *except*

A.  The Beck Depression Inventory (BDI) is not useful in the assessment of depression in Parkinson's disease, because the physical symptoms of Parkinson's disease affect the interpretation of the BDI.
B.  Depression in Parkinson's disease is a major determinant of quality of life, more so than the severity of the motor impairment or the effects of medications.
C.  Poststroke depression increases the mortality rate at 1 year after stroke.
D.  Late-life-onset depression and "depressive pseudodementia" confer an increased risk of eventual diagnosis of dementia of the Alzheimer's type.
E.  Dementia of the Alzheimer's type, when complicated by depression, is associated with an increased rate of nursing home placement, decline in activities of daily living (ADLs), and cognitive decline.

**The correct response is option A.**

The BDI is useful for assessment of depression in Parkinson's disease, despite the overlap of somatic items with symptoms of Parkinson's disease.

   Depression in Parkinson's disease (present in approximately 50% of Parkinson's patients) is a major determinant of quality-of-life ratings, exceeding the effects of both disease severity and medication. Poststroke depression is associated with a heightened risk of mortality 1 year and 10 years after the stroke. Late-onset depression and pseudodementia with depression are highly correlated with the eventual diagnosis of Alzheimer's dementia. In Alzheimer's dementia, depression is associated with more adverse outcomes, such as nursing home placement, decline in ADLs, more rapid cognitive decline, and increased mortality. **(pp. 202–203)**

9.5    Selective serotonin reuptake inhibitors (SSRIs) are useful for treatment of major depression in the medically ill. Controlled trials have demonstrated benefit of SSRIs for depression in all of the following illnesses *except*

A.  Cardiac disease.
B.  Stroke.
C.  Cancer.
D.  HIV.
E.  Parkinson's disease.

**The correct response is option E.**

Although no controlled trials of SSRIs in Parkinson's disease have been conducted, open trials have indicated that SSRIs may improve depressive symptoms in patients with Parkinson's disease. **(p. 205)**

9.6    Which of the following novel antidepressants is *most* likely to rapidly alleviate insomnia and anorexia in cancer patients?

    A   Moclobemide.
    B.  Venlafaxine.
    C.  Bupropion.
    D.  Mirtazapine.
    E.  Nefazodone.

**The correct response is option D.**

Of the novel antidepressants listed, mirtazapine is the most likely to improve insomnia and anorexia in medically ill patients, because its main side effects are sedation and weight gain (Stimmel et al. 1997).

Moclobemide is efficacious in reducing depressive symptoms in patients with Alzheimer's disease. Extended-release venlafaxine has been found to be effective in breast cancer patients with hot flashes (Loprinzi et al. 2000) and in patients with neuropathic pain (Davis and Smith 1999; Dwight et al. 1998). Bupropion may be useful in treating patients with prominent fatigue, and nefazodone has been found effective in open trials with HIV patients (Elliot et al. 1999). **(p. 206)**

# References

Berkman LF, Blumenthal J, Burg M, et al: Effects of treating depression and low perceived social support on clinical events after myocardial infarction: the Enhancing Recovery in Coronary Heart Disease Patients (ENRICHD). JAMA 289:3106–3116, 2003

Davis JL, Smith RL: Painful peripheral diabetic neuropathy treated with venlafaxine HCl extended release capsules. Diabetes Care 22:1909–1910, 1999

Dwight MM, Arnold LM, O'Brien H, et al: An open clinical trial of venlafaxine treatment of fibromyalgia. Psychosomatics 39:14–17, 1998

Elliot AJ, Russo J, Bergam K, et al: Antidepressant efficacy in HIV-seropositive outpatients with major depressive disorder: an open trial of nefazodone. J Clin Psychiatry 60:226–231, 1999

Glassman AH, O'Connor CM, Califf RM, et al: Sertraline treatment of major depression in patients with acute MI or unstable angina. JAMA 288:701–709, 2002

Loprinzi CL, Kugler JW, Sloan JA, et al: Venlafaxine in management of hot flashes in survivors of breast cancer: a randomized controlled trial. Lancet 356:2059–2063, 2000

Stimmel GL, Dopheide JA, Stahl SM: Mirtazapine: an antidepressant with noradrenergic and specific serotonergic effects. Pharmacotherapy 17:10–21, 1997

# C H A P T E R  1 0

# Suicidality

*Select the single best response for each question.*

10.1 Which of the following statements concerning completed suicide is *true*?

A. The known suicide rate in 2001 was twice as high as it was in 1900.
B. Between 1990 and 2001, suicide rates increased in every age category.
C. In 2001, annual suicide rates per 100,000 individuals increased throughout the life span from childhood to old age.
D. The suicide rate among women is three times higher than that among men.
E. In 2001, white Americans killed themselves at less than half the rate of nonwhite Americans.

**The correct response is option C.**

In 2001, annual suicide rates per 100,000 individuals increased throughout the life span.
   The known suicide rate in 2001 was nearly identical to what it was in 1900. Between 1990 and 2001, suicide rates have decreased in every age category. The suicide rate among women is three times *lower* than that among men. Nonwhite Americans killed themselves at less than half the rate of white Americans in 2001. **(p. 221)**

10.2 In general, patients who attempted suicide, in comparison with those who died by suicide,

A. Did not have long-standing mental illness.
B. Did not have carefully considered plans.
C. Did not have command hallucinations.
D. Were not ruminative about their suicide intent.
E. All of the above.

**The correct response is option E.**

All of the above statements are true. In a study by Hall et al. (1999), suicide attempters in general did not have carefully considered plans, long-standing mental illness, command hallucinations, or particular ruminations about their suicidal intent. **(p. 222)**

10.3 It has been repeatedly shown in general-population studies conducted in the United States and Europe that the vast majority of completed suicides are associated with

A. Depression.
B. Schizophrenia.
C. Alcoholism.
D. A and C.
E. A and B.

**The correct response is option D.**

According to repeated studies, depression and alcoholism are the psychiatric illnesses associated with the vast majority of completed suicides. **(p. 221)**

10.4 Which of the following statements concerning suicide in medically ill patients is *false*?

A. The majority of terminally ill cancer patients have a high desire for hastened death.
B. Suicides in the medically ill appear to be related to unrecognized comorbid psychiatric illnesses.
C. The will to live in terminally ill patients may be best predicted by presence and severity of depression; anxiety; shortness of breath; and sense of well-being.
D. Cancer patients who die by suicide are psychiatrically similar to noncancer patients who commit suicide.
E. Most patients who decide to stop dialysis are not influenced by major depression or suicidal ideation.

**The correct response is option A.**

In a study by Breitbart et al. (2000), only 17% of terminally ill cancer patients had a high desire for hastened death.

Suicides in the medically ill appear to be related to frequently unrecognized depression, substance-related disorders, delirium, dementia, and personality disorder. The will to live in the terminally ill fluctuates and is mostly predicted by depression, anxiety, shortness of breath, and sense of well-being. **(pp. 226–227)**

Most patients who decide to stop dialysis do not seem to be influenced by major depression. **(p. 237)**

10.5 With regard to physician-assisted suicide, the United States Supreme Court in 1997 ruled that

A. There is a constitutional right to physician-assisted suicide.
B. States can prohibit physician conduct in which the primary purpose is to hasten death.
C. States cannot enact legislation that allows physician-assisted suicide.
D. All of the above.
E. None of the above.

**The correct response is option B.**

The United States Supreme Court ruled in 1997 that there is no constitutional right to physician-assisted suicide and that states can prohibit physician conduct in which the primary purpose is to hasten death (Burt 1997). States, however, can enact legislation that allows physician-assisted suicide (e.g., Oregon's Death With Dignity Act). **(p. 229)**

# References

Breitbart W, Rosenfeld B, Pessin H, et al: Depression, hopelessness, and desire for hastened death in terminally ill patients with cancer. JAMA 284:2907–2911, 2000

Burt R: The Supreme Court speaks—not assisted suicide but a constitutional right to palliative care. N Engl J Med 337:1234–1236, 1997

Hall R, Platt D, Hall R: Suicide risk assessment: a review of risk factors for suicide in 100 patients who made severe suicide attempts. Psychosomatics 40:18–27, 1999

# CHAPTER 11

# Mania, Catatonia, and Psychosis

*Select the single best response for each question.*

11.1 It may be difficult to differentiate secondary mania from delirium in the acutely ill patient, because many of the presenting symptoms overlap. Which of the following symptoms is more suggestive of secondary mania than of delirium?

  A. Waxing and waning course.
  B. Variable level of consciousness.
  C. Visual hallucinations.
  D. Pressured speech.
  E. Visual illusions.

**The correct response is option D.**

Delirium differs from secondary mania in its waxing and waning course, clouding of consciousness, and visual hallucinations and illusions, whereas secondary mania is suggested by manic affect, hypersexuality, and pressured speech. **(p. 236)**

11.2 Secondary mania may be either transient or relatively persistent, depending in substantial part on the putative etiological agent or condition. Which of the following would more likely be associated with transient/reversible rather than persistent secondary mania?

  A. Traumatic brain injury.
  B. Stroke.
  C. Dopamine agonists.
  D. Neoplasm.
  E. Multiple sclerosis.

**The correct response is option C.**

Cases of secondary mania caused by psychostimulants or dopamine agonists typically are totally reversible, whereas symptoms may persist in patients with mania secondary to central nervous system (CNS) injury, a neoplasm, infection, or an underlying neurodegenerative disease. **(pp. 236–237)**

11.3 Endocrine disturbances and substances of abuse are associated with secondary mania. All of the following statements are true *except*

  A. Hyperthyroidism may cause mania.
  B. Hypothyroidism may cause mania.
  C. Depression is more common following systemic use of corticosteroids than is mania.
  D. Psychotic symptoms have been reported in 50% of hypomanic or depressive episodes following corticosteroid use.
  E. Hypothyroidism induces rapid cycling in established bipolar disorder patients.

**The correct response is option B.**

Hypothyroidism does not in itself cause mania, but it is well known to induce rapid cycling in patients with primary bipolar disorder. **(p. 239)**

11.4    Core features of catatonia include all of the following symptoms or signs *except*

    A. Stupor.
    B. Motoric immobility.
    C. Mutism.
    D. Catalepsy.
    E. Auditory hallucinations.

**The correct response is option E.**

Auditory hallucinations are not present in catatonia. The core features of catatonia are stupor, motoric immobility, mutism, negativism, excitement, catalepsy, and posturing. These features are the same regardless of whether the condition occurs in the context of a mood, psychotic, or medical state. **(p. 240)**

11.5    Patients with seizure disorders commonly have comorbid psychiatric illness. Notably, psychotic symptoms are a significant problem that may complicate diagnosis and management. All of the following are true *except*

    A. Psychotic symptoms are most common during the interictal phase.
    B. Psychotic symptoms are most common with evidence of left-sided seizure foci or temporal lobe lesions.
    C. Psychotic symptoms associated with nonconvulsive status epilepticus are more common with partial complex seizures.
    D. Postictal psychotic symptoms typically occur immediately following a seizure.
    E. Postictal psychosis follows an increase in seizure frequency.

**The correct response is option D.**

Postictal psychosis follows an increase in the frequency of seizures, usually with a nonpsychotic period of 1–7 days between the last seizure and the psychosis. **(pp. 243–244)**

11.6    Psychotic symptoms may occur in patients with kidney disease and require treatment. Which of the following antipsychotics require dosage modification when used in patients with renal failure?

    A. Ziprasidone.
    B. Olanzapine.
    C. Haloperidol.
    D. Clozapine.
    E. Risperidone.

**The correct response is option E.**

In renal failure, clearance of risperidone is decreased; therefore, risperidone should be started at lower doses than usual, and dose increases should be gradual. **(p. 246)**

# CHAPTER 12

# Anxiety Disorders

*Select the single best response for each question.*

12.1    A recent meta-analysis identified five variables that correlate with higher rates of panic disorder among individuals seeking treatment for chest pain in emergency rooms. All of the following variables were identified *except*

A.  Absence of coronary artery disease.
B.  Atypical quality of chest pain.
C.  Male gender.
D.  Younger age.
E.  High level of self-reported anxiety.

**The correct response is option C.**

Male gender is not a variable that correlates with higher rates of panic disorder.

   In a recent meta-analysis, Huffman and Pollack (2003) identified five variables that correlate with higher rates of panic disorder among individuals seeking treatment for chest pain in emergency rooms or cardiology clinics: 1) absence of coronary artery disease, 2) atypical quality of chest pain, 3) female sex, 4) younger age, and 5) a high level of self-reported anxiety. **(p. 252)**

12.2    A life-threatening illness, such as cancer, is a stressor that can precipitate posttraumatic stress disorder (PTSD). However, this trauma is different from more usual PTSD stressors in which of the following ways?

A.  The threat is external.
B.  The principal stressor relates to the fear of recurrence.
C.  The ongoing stressor is the memory of past events.
D.  The threat arises from one's own body.
E.  B and D.

**The correct response is option E.**

Life-threatening illness such as cancer is a stressor that can precipitate PTSD (Kangas et al. 2002; Smith et al. 1999). However, this trauma is different from more usual PTSD stressors such as rape in two principal ways: 1) the threat arises from one's own body, and 2) once the patient has been treated, the ongoing stressor is often not the memory of past events but rather the fear of recurrence (Green et al. 1997). **(p. 253)**

12.3    Regarding therapies that have been found effective in reducing anxiety and physical symptoms in medically ill patients, which of the following statements is *false*?

A.  Muscular conditions such as tension headaches respond better to more cognitive techniques.
B.  Migraine headaches respond better to autogenic training.
C.  Relaxation techniques have been used to reduce pain in patients with chronic pain.

D. Guided imagery with relaxation has been shown to be an effective technique for reducing anxiety.
E. Musculoskeletal disorders may respond better to muscle relaxation.

**The correct response is option A.**

Muscular conditions such as tension headaches and musculoskeletal disorders may respond better to muscle relaxation; migraine headaches and hypertension, to autogenic training; and anxieties and phobias, to more cognitive techniques; however, further research is needed (Lehrer et al. 1994).

When used by a skilled practitioner with a patient who is open to the approach, all of these techniques may be helpful in reducing symptoms of various conditions exacerbated by anxiety and stress. Guided imagery with relaxation and hypnosis has also been an effective technique to reduce anxiety (Payne and Massie 2000). Relaxation techniques have been used to decrease the use of medications in hypertensive patients, to decrease pain in patients with chronic pain, and to expedite recovery and decrease complications in postsurgical patients (Benson 1988). **(p. 261)**

12.4 Advantages of selective serotonin reuptake inhibitors (SSRIs) in treating anxiety disorders in medically ill patients include all of the following *except*

A. SSRIs do not produce cardiac conduction problems.
B. SSRIs do not cause orthostatic hypotension.
C. SSRIs do not lead to physical dependence.
D. SSRIs do not produce sexual dysfunction.
E. SSRIs have few side effects.

**The correct response is option D.**

One of the main drawbacks of SSRI use is a genuine high incidence of sexual dysfunction in both men and women. However, these medications have few side effects and therefore are generally quite safe for the medically ill; they do not result in cardiac conduction problems, orthostatic hypotension, or physical dependence. **(p. 263)**

12.5 Regarding the use of beta-adrenergic blockers to treat anxiety symptoms, which of the following statements is *true*?

A. Beta-blockers are most efficacious in treating panic disorder.
B. Beta-blockers work best when used in specific anxiety-producing situations.
C. Beta-blockers are the treatment of choice for anxiety in chronic obstructive pulmonary disease (COPD) patients.
D. Patients with insulin-dependent diabetes should be prescribed nonselective beta-blockers.
E. Beta-blockers can improve peripheral vascular disease.

**The correct response is option B.**

Beta-adrenergic blockers produce anxiolytic effects by blocking autonomic hyperarousal (elevated pulse, elevated blood pressure, sweating tremors) associated with anxiety responses. They work best when used for specific anxiety-producing situations, such as performance anxiety and public speaking; they are less efficacious for panic disorder and social phobias. All beta-blockers are contraindicated in persons with asthma or COPD, and they can worsen peripheral vascular disease (Barnes 2000). Patients with insulin-dependent diabetes should not be prescribed nonselective beta-blockers; because those medications block the sympathetic nervous system response to hypoglycemia, the patient may be unaware of symptoms and may be less likely to respond appropriately (Kaplan 2001). **(p. 265)**

# References

Barnes PJ: Airway pharmacology, in Textbook of Respiratory Medicine, 3rd Edition. Edited by Murray JF, Nadel JA. Philadelphia, PA, WB Saunders, 2000, pp 267–296

Benson H: The relaxation response: a bridge between medicine and religion. Harv Ment Health Lett 4 (March):4–6, 1988

Green BL, Epstein SA, Krupnick JL, et al: Trauma and medical illness: assessing trauma-related disorders in medical settings, in Assessing Psychological Trauma and PTSD. Edited by Wilson JP, Keane TM. New York, Guilford, 1997, pp 160–191

Huffman JC, Pollack MH: Predicting panic disorder among patients with chest pain: an analysis of the literature. Psychosomatics 44:222–236, 2003

Kangas M, Henry JL, Bryant RA: Posttraumatic stress disorder following cancer: a conceptual and empirical review. Clin Psychol Rev 22:499–524, 2002

Kaplan N: Systemic hypertension: therapy, in Heart Disease: A Textbook of Cardiovascular Medicine, 6th Edition. Edited by Braunwald E, Zipes DP, Libby P. Philadelphia, PA, WB Saunders, 2001, pp 27–28

Lehrer PM, Carr R, Sargunaraj D, et al: Stress management techniques: are they all equivalent, or do they have specific effects? Biofeedback Self Regul 19:353–401, 1994

Payne D, Massie MJ: Anxiety in palliative care, in Handbook of Psychiatry in Palliative Medicine. Edited by Chochinov HM, Breitbart W. New York, Oxford University Press, 2000, pp 63–74

Smith MY, Redd WH, Peyser C, et al: Post-traumatic stress disorder in cancer: a review. Psychooncology 8:521–537, 1999

# CHAPTER 13

# Somatization and Somatoform Disorders

*Select the single best response for each question.*

13.1 The more general concept of somatization (bridging several of the somatoform disorders) may be used as an explanatory model for many behaviors presenting in the physically ill patient. Which of the following statements is *true*?

A. Somatization is best understood as a defense against the acknowledgment of a psychiatric disorder.
B. Fifty percent or more of depressed patients in primary care clinics manifest predominantly somatic complaints.
C. Somatic symptoms in depression are related to mood symptoms alone, not to concurrent anxiety.
D. Although somatization is common in panic disorder, hypochondriacal fears of a specific illness are not.
E. Somatization in schizophrenia is unrelated to high levels of "expressed emotion" in family members.

**The correct response is option B.**

It is estimated that 50% or more of patients presenting to primary care clinics with major depressive disorder do so with predominantly somatic complaints rather than with cognitive or affective symptoms of depression (Simon and Gureje 1999).

Somatization is not a defense against acknowledging the presence of a psychiatric disorder. Somatic symptoms in depression are related to concomitant anxiety, the tendency to amplify somatic distress, and difficulty identifying and communicating emotional distress. Somatization and hypochondriasis are common among patients with panic disorder, particularly panic with agoraphobia. Somatization in schizophrenia is associated with expressed emotion within families, emotional distress, and medication side effects. **(pp. 273–275)**

13.2 Various pathophysiological mechanisms have been employed to provide explanatory models for somatization. These include several physiological, psychological, and interpersonal mechanisms. Which of the following would be considered a physiological (as opposed to a psychological) mechanism?

A. Cerebral information processing.
B. Perceptual factors.
C. Beliefs.
D. Mood.
E. Personality factors.

**The correct response is option A.**

Cerebral information processing is a physiological mechanism of somatization. Perceptual factors, beliefs, mood, and personality factors are psychological mechanisms. **(p. 275, Table 13–2)**

13.3    The clinical management of somatization is best accomplished along several dimensions, and the psychosomatic medicine consultant may be of help to colleagues in effectuating such management plans. Three possible management approaches—reattribution, psychotherapeutic, and directive—to the patient with somatization disorder have been described. All of the following are true *except*

A.  The reattribution approach seeks to link physical symptoms to psychological factors in the patient's life.
B.  The psychotherapeutic approach focuses on the centrality of the relationship between patient and physician.
C.  The directive approach frames the somatization behavior as a medical problem, and interventions are made in a medical context.
D.  The psychotherapeutic approach is preferred for openly hostile patients who deny psychological factors in their symptoms.
E.  The reattribution approach is useful in medical inpatient settings with reasonably insightful patients.

**The correct response is option D.**

The psychotherapeutic approach is most suitable for patients with persistent somatization who are willing to explore the effects of psychosocial factors on their symptoms. The directive approach is most useful for hostile patients who deny the importance of psychological or social factors in their symptomatology. The reattribution approach helps the patient to link physical symptoms with psychological or stressful factors. **(p. 278)**

13.4    In regard to the clinical features of somatization disorder, all of the following are true *except*

A.  Symptoms begin before the age of 30 years, often during the teens.
B.  Depression, substance abuse, and antisocial personality disorder are common in first-degree relatives of somatization disorder patients.
C.  Women with somatization disorder are less likely to have a history of sexual abuse than are women with primary major depression.
D.  Patients present their histories in a vague yet dramatic and colorful manner.
E.  The majority of somatization disorder patients have psychiatric comorbidity.

**The correct response is option C.**

Women with somatization disorder are more likely to have a history of sexual abuse than are women with primary mood disorders.
    Up to 75% of patients with somatization disorder have a comorbid Axis I diagnosis.
**(pp. 280–281)**

13.5    Which of the following is *not* among the most common comorbid psychiatric conditions in somatization disorder?

A.  Obsessive-compulsive disorder.
B.  Major depression.
C.  Dysthymic disorder.
D.  Panic disorder.
E.  Simple phobia.

**The correct response is option A.**

The most common comorbid psychiatric diagnoses in somatization disorder are major depressive disorder, dysthymic disorder, panic disorder, simple phobia, and substance abuse. **(p. 281)**

13.6  Conversion disorder is a somatoform disorder that often has an acute and dramatic presentation. Which of the following is *not* true of conversion disorder?

    A. Presentations include pseudoseizures, ataxia, and sensory deficits.
    B. Social settings with substantial secondary gain increase the likelihood of conversion disorder.
    C. A relationship with childhood abuse is especially common in pseudoseizure conversion patients.
    D. Higher rates of conversion disorder are found in highly developed nations.
    E. The paradoxical emotional response of *la belle indifference* does not confer prognostic significance.

**The correct response is option D.**

Much higher rates of conversion disorder have been described in developing countries and in isolated rural American settings.
    Paralysis, pseudoseizures, amnesia, ataxia, and blindness are common in conversion disorder. Settings such as military combat have increased rates of conversion. **(pp. 282–283)**

13.7  Patients with hypochondriasis can lead a physician to pursue an extensive diagnostic workup. Which of the following statements is *true*?

    A. Onset of hypochondriasis is most common in middle or late middle age.
    B. Hypochondriasis patients accept that good health can involve minor symptoms.
    C. Psychiatric comorbidity in hypochondriasis includes generalized anxiety disorder, major depression, and panic disorder.
    D. Because of their fear of "legitimate" medical illness, patients with hypochondriasis are unlikely to use alternative health care practices.
    E. Presence of a "real" comorbid medical illness is associated with a worse prognosis.

**The correct response is option C.**

Patients with hypochondriasis have a high rate of psychiatric comorbidity, with the most common comorbid diagnoses being generalized anxiety disorder, dysthymia, major depressive disorder, somatization disorder, and panic disorder.
    Onset of hypochondriasis is most common in early adulthood. Patients with hypochondriasis believe that good health is a relatively symptom-free state. These patients often seek out complementary health care services. Positive prognostic features in hypochondriasis include presence of a comorbid medical condition, acute onset, brief duration, mild symptoms, absence of secondary gain, and absence of psychiatric comorbidity. **(pp. 284–285)**

# Reference

Simon GE, Gureje O: Stability of somatization disorder and somatization symptoms among primary care patients. Arch Gen Psychiatry 56:90–95, 1999

# C H A P T E R   1 4

# Deception Syndromes: Factitious Disorders and Malingering

*Select the single best response for each question.*

14.1 Regarding simulated physical diseases, which of the following statements are *true*?

A. Somatoform disorders are considered to be of unconscious etiology.
B. Factitious disorders are considered to be of conscious production and unconscious motivation.
C. Malingering is considered to be of conscious production and motivation.
D. All of the above.
E. None of the above.

**The correct response is option D.**

In the current diagnostic classification of DSM-IV-TR (American Psychiatric Association 2000), simulated diseases, such as somatization disorder, are placed within the category of somatoform disorders. These disorders are considered to be of unconscious etiology. Factitious disorders, considered to be of conscious production but of unconscious motivation, are included among Axis I diagnoses in a separate category. Malingering, considered to be of both conscious production and conscious motivation, is assigned a V code (other conditions that may be a focus of clinical attention). **(p. 297)**

14.2 Classic Munchausen syndrome includes all of the following essential components *except*

A. Travel from hospital to hospital.
B. Simulation of disease.
C. Unconscious self-induction of disease.
D. Pseudologia fantastica.
E. Use of aliases to disguise identity.

**The correct response is option C.**

Classic Munchausen syndrome consists of three essential components: 1) the simulation or self-induction of disease; 2) pseudologia fantastica; and 3) travel from hospital to hospital, often using aliases to disguise identity. These patients frequently present to the emergency room with dramatic symptoms such as hemoptysis, acute chest pain suggestive of a myocardial infarction, or coma from self-induced hypoglycemia. **(p. 299)**

14.3 Patients with factitious disorder

A. Often have a Cluster B personality disorder.
B. Commonly have an Axis I disorder, especially schizophrenia.

C. Have a need to be the center of attention.

D. All of the above.

E. A and C.

**The correct response is option E.**

The large majority of patients with factitious disorder have an underlying severe personality disorder, usually of the Cluster B type, and they need to feel that they are the center of attention. Factitious behavior can be seen as a form of acting-out, similar to other acting-out behaviors observed in Cluster B personality disorders.

Axis I comorbidity, including major depression and schizophrenia, has been described in factitious disorder but is not common. However, it must be kept in mind that psychiatric symptoms may also be simulated by these patients. **(p. 301)**

14.4    In studies of families with Munchausen syndrome by proxy, investigators have found all of the following commonly observed features except

A. A dominant and aggressive husband and a caretaking and supportive wife.

B. Intense family–group loyalty, with little protective concern for the child.

C. A multigenerational pattern of abnormal illness behavior.

D. Enmeshment of parent–child relationships.

E. None of the above.

**The correct response is option A.**

Studies of families with Munchausen syndrome by proxy have revealed that the wife tends to be more dominant and aggressive, whereas the husband is more caretaking and supportive.

In studies by Griffith (1988), commonly observed features were 1) enmeshment of parent–child relationships; 2) multigenerational themes of dominance and submission in parent–child relationships; 3) intense family–group loyalty, with little protective concern for the needs of the developing child; and 4) a multigenerational pattern of abnormal illness behavior on the maternal side of the family. **(p. 304)**

14.5    The form of malingering most frequently encountered by psychosomatic medicine specialists is

A. Falsification of laboratory reports.

B. Production of new illness.

C. Contamination of laboratory samples.

D. Embellishment of a previous or concurrent illness.

E. None of the above.

**The correct response is option D.**

Embellishment of previous or concurrent illness is probably the form of malingering most frequently encountered by psychosomatic subspecialists. Malingering symptoms fall into four major categories: 1) production or simulation of an illness, 2) exacerbation of a previous illness, 3) exaggeration of symptoms, and 4) falsification of laboratory samples or laboratory reports. **(p. 305)**

# References

American Psychiatric Association: Diagnostic and Statistical Manual of Mental Disorders, 4th Edition, Text Revision. Washington, DC, American Psychiatric Association, 2000

Griffith JL: The family systems of Munchausen syndrome by proxy. Fam Process 27:423–437, 1988

# C H A P T E R 1 5

# Eating Disorders

*Select the single best response for each question.*

15.1 Eating disorders are among the most challenging psychiatric illnesses in practice and are associated with much psychiatric and medical comorbidity. Which of the following statements is *true*?

A. Anorexia nervosa and bulimia nervosa are associated with a 5% mortality rate per decade of illness.
B. Despite their lack of clinical eating disorders, semistarvation research subjects exhibited ritualistic behaviors similar to those of anorexia nervosa patients.
C. Eating binges in bulimia nervosa feature foods composed primarily of carbohydrates.
D. Most bulimia nervosa patients who seek treatment are overweight or obese.
E. Progression from restricting anorexia nervosa to bulimia nervosa and normal-weight bulimia nervosa to anorexia nervosa are both quite common, about 50%.

**The correct response is option B.**

In the 1948 Minnesota semistarvation study (Franklin et al. 1948), subjects exhibited ritualistic behaviors similar to those seen in anorexia nervosa, suggesting that these features might be driven by the physiological effects of starvation.

Whereas anorexia nervosa is associated with a 5% mortality rate per decade of illness, bulimia nervosa is much less lethal. Eating binges in bulimia nervosa do not primarily involve carbohydrates. Most bulimic patients who seek treatment are not overweight. The progression from anorexia nervosa to bulimia nervosa is quite common (50% in patients with restricting anorexia nervosa), whereas the progression from normal-weight bulimia nervosa to anorexia nervosa is much less frequent.
**(pp. 311–312)**

15.2 Among the following illnesses in children, which is considered a feeding disorder rather than an eating disorder?

A. Food avoidance emotional disorder.
B. Pervasive refusal syndrome.
C. Selective eating.
D. Functional dysphagia.
E. Pica.

**The correct response is option E.**

Pica is considered a feeding disorder, whereas food avoidance emotional disorder, selective eating, pervasive refusal syndrome, functional dysphagia, and full-syndrome anorexia nervosa are eating disorders that may occur before puberty. **(p. 314)**

15.3 Regarding the epidemiology and course of eating disorders, which of the following statements is *true?*

A. Anorexia nervosa and bulimia nervosa are equally prevalent in young women, seen in about 1%–2%.
B. Epidemiological evidence strongly supports significant recent increases in the prevalence of both anorexia nervosa and bulimia nervosa.
C. Anorexia nervosa patients treated during adolescence have a more favorable long-term outcome than do those treated later in life.
D. Among bulimia nervosa patients, less than 10% practice bingeing and purging 10 years after initial presentation.
E. Anorexia nervosa patients with obsessive-compulsive personality traits have a better prognosis than do those with histrionic personality traits.

**The correct response is option C.**

Patients with anorexia nervosa treated during adolescence appear to have more favorable long-term outcomes.

Anorexia nervosa has a prevalence of 0.7% among teenage girls, whereas bulimia nervosa is more prevalent (about 1%–2%). The evidence of an increase in bulimia nervosa over the past few decades is considerably stronger than the evidence of an increase in anorexia nervosa. Nearly one-third of patients with bulimia nervosa continue to practice bingeing and purging 10 years after presentation. Patients with histrionic personality traits have a better prognosis than do those with obsessive-compulsive personality traits. **(pp. 315–316)**

15.4 Laboratory tests that should be routinely performed in eating disorder patients include all of the following *except*

A. Serum electrolytes.
B. Blood urea nitrogen and creatinine.
C. Thyroid function tests.
D. Complete blood cell count.
E. Serum amylase.

**The correct response is option E.**

Serum amylase, luteinizing hormone, and follicle-stimulating hormone levels are not gathered routinely.

Routine workups include serum electrolytes, blood urea nitrogen and creatinine, liver enzymes, serum albumin, thyroid function tests, complete blood cell count, and urinalysis. Severely malnourished patients should receive an electrocardiogram and have their calcium magnesium and phosphate levels checked. **(p. 317)**

15.5 Psychopharmacological approaches to eating disorders may have an important adjunctive role in treatment. Which of the following statements is *false?*

A. For bulimia nervosa, all classes of antidepressants are effective.
B. Fluoxetine is the only U.S. Food and Drug Administration (FDA)–approved antidepressant for bulimia nervosa.
C. Medications alone have not been shown to produce long-term remission.
D. In general, patients with anorexia nervosa do not respond well to pharmacotherapy.

E. Olanzapine is a promising agent for treatment of anorexia nervosa solely because of its effect on appetite and weight gain, and it has been shown to be effective in controlled trials.

**The correct response is option E.**

Olanzapine may be useful in the treatment of anorexia nervosa because of its ability to target the delusions, anxiety, and obsessions that often afflict anorexic patients and for its documented side effect of weight gain. However, double-blind, randomized trials are necessary before firm conclusions can be drawn about this agent's efficacy. **(p. 327)**

15.6   The most widely studied psychotherapy model for eating disorders is

    A. Psychoanalysis.
    B. Psychodynamic psychotherapy.
    C. Cognitive-behavioral therapy (CBT).
    D. Interpersonal psychotherapy.
    E. Supportive psychotherapy.

**The correct response is option C.**

CBT is the most widely studied method of psychotherapy for eating disorders, because it targets cognitive disturbances and behavioral aspects of eating. Most studies of CBT for eating disorders have examined patients with bulimia nervosa. **(pp. 327–328)**

# Reference

Franklin JC, Schiele BC, Brozek J, et al: Observations of human behavior in experimental semistarvation and rehabilitation. J Clin Psychol 4:28–45, 1948

# CHAPTER 16

# Sleep Disorders

*Select the single best response for each question.*

16.1 Which of the following are polysomnographic characteristics of stage III/IV sleep in healthy individuals?

A. Spindles.
B. Slow eye movements.
C. K complexes.
D. Slow electroencephalogram (EEG) frequency.
E. A and C.

**The correct response is option D.**

Stage III/IV sleep in healthy adults is characterized by slow EEG frequency.

Spindles and K complexes are characteristic of stage II sleep, whereas slow eye movements are characteristic of stage I sleep. **(p. 336, Table 16–1)**

16.2 Regarding narcolepsy, which of the following statements is *true*?

A. In one U.S. community sample, narcolepsy was found to have a prevalence of 0.8%.
B. Narcolepsy is more common in women.
C. Narcolepsy is believed to be primarily a familial disease.
D. Narcolepsy commonly starts during the fourth decade of life.
E. Approximately 65% of patients with narcolepsy have cataplexy.

**The correct response is option E.**

In the U.S. community sample studied by Silber et al. (2001), 64% of narcolepsy patients were found to have cataplexy.

In that same sample, narcolepsy was observed to have a prevalence of 0.06% (Silber et al. 2001). Incidence data from the same study confirmed the long-standing impression that narcolepsy is slightly more common in men (1.72 per 100,000) than in women (1.05 per 100,000). The disease most commonly starts during the second decade of life and is a chronic condition. Narcolepsy is no longer believed to be a familial disease, although a small number of affected families have been identified (Overeem et al. 2001). **(p. 339)**

16.3 Symptoms of narcolepsy include

A. Excessive daytime sleepiness.
B. Sleep paralysis.
C. Episodic sleep attacks.
D. Cataplexy.
E. All of the above.

**The correct response is option E.**

Narcolepsy is characterized by chronic excessive daytime sleepiness with episodic sleep attacks. Approximately 65%–75% of patients with narcolepsy have cataplexy (a condition in which an emotional trigger, most commonly laughter, provokes abrupt muscle atonia without loss of consciousness). Other associated symptoms of narcolepsy include sleep paralysis and hypnagogic and hypnopompic hallucinations (vivid dreaming occurring at the time of sleep onset and awakening that can be difficult to distinguish from reality). Disturbed nocturnal sleep has been added as a fifth part of this constellation of symptoms. (p. 340)

16.4    Essential signs and symptoms of obstructive sleep apnea are

A. Excessive daytime sleepiness.
B. Snoring.
C. Obstructed breathing during sleep.
D. A and C.
E. A, B, and C.

**The correct response is option D.**

Excessive daytime sleepiness and obstructed breathing during sleep are essential signs and symptoms of obstructive sleep apnea. Although essentially all patients with obstructive sleep apnea snore, all persons who snore do not have obstructive sleep apnea. Snoring is an extremely common phenomenon, affecting 25% of men and 15% of women. For this reason, screening for obstructive sleep apnea must rely on more than simply a history of snoring. (p. 342)

16.5    Regarding restless legs syndrome, which of the following statements is *false*?

A. The overall prevalence rate is estimated to be between 5% and 10%.
B. It is more common in older individuals.
C. Symptoms are worsened by activity.
D. It may occur in association with anemia.
E. It can develop during the third trimester of pregnancy.

**The correct response is option C.**

Lack of exercise, together with nicotine dependence, diabetes mellitus, and high body mass index, increases the risk of restless legs syndrome.

The overall prevalence of restless legs syndrome is 10%, with equal rates in men and women, although the condition is more prominent in older individuals. Restless legs syndrome sometimes occurs in association with anemia and iron deficiency and can develop during the third trimester of pregnancy, most likely because of the presence of functional anemia. (p. 345)

# References

Overeem S, Mignot E, Gert van Dijk J, et al: Narcolepsy: clinical features, new pathophysiologic insights, and future perspectives. J Clin Neurophysiol 18:78–105, 2001

Silber M, Krahn L, Olson E, et al: Epidemiology of narcolepsy in Olmsted County, Minnesota: a population-based study. Sleep 24 (abstract suppl):A98, 2001

# C H A P T E R   1 7

# Sexual Disorders

*Select the single best response for each question.*

17.1 Sexual function in heart disease patients may be an important determinant of quality of life, thus affecting psychiatric status. All of the following statements are true *except*

  A. Sexual activity decreases and perception of sexual dysfunction increases after myocardial infarction (MI).
  B. Resumption of sexual intercourse with the usual partner and in the usual setting after MI does not affect cardiac morbidity.
  C. Decreased ejection fraction is associated with reduced libido and impaired sexual performance.
  D. Increasing exercise, losing weight, stopping smoking, and decreasing alcohol use all have been shown to reduce erectile dysfunction in cardiac patients.
  E. Sildenafil is safe and effective in stable angina if nitrates are avoided.

**The correct response is option D.**

Increasing exercise reduced the risk of erectile dysfunction in cardiac patients, but weight loss, cessation of smoking, and reduction of alcohol use did not. **(pp. 360–361)**

17.2 Sexual function may be adversely affected by several oncological interventions. Which of the following statements is *true*?

  A. Gynecological surgery for cancer typically results in a dramatic loss of sexual function.
  B. Decline in sexual function following prostate cancer treatment is attributable to erectile dysfunction, as libido and orgasmic function are usually unaffected.
  C. Sildenafil has been shown to be effective for erectile dysfunction after $^{125}$I seed implantation radiotherapy.
  D. In testicular cancer, sexual performance concerns far outweigh concerns about retrograde ejaculation and infertility.
  E. Intramuscular androgens are not effective in treating sexual dysfunction following bilateral orchiectomy for testicular cancer.

**The correct response is option C.**

Sildenafil improved erections in 74% of men with erectile dysfunction following $^{125}$I seed implantation radiotherapy.

Marked deterioration in sexual functioning after gynecological oncological surgery has not been typical. Following treatment for prostate cancer, men are as distressed about loss of desire and anorgasmia as they are about erectile dysfunction. In testicular cancer, concerns about performance are less prominent than concerns about retrograde ejaculation and infertility. Intramuscular androgens are effective in treating sexual dysfunction following bilateral orchiectomy for testicular cancer. **(p. 362)**

17.3 Sexual function may be a major concern for diabetic patients, and this area must be addressed in the context of other complications. All of the following statements are true *except*

A. Erectile dysfunction in diabetic men correlates with increased levels of glycosylated hemoglobin.
B. Depression in diabetes is associated with sexual dysfunction and other diabetic complications.
C. Sexual dysfunction in diabetic men is typically limited to erectile dysfunction.
D. Depression can produce abnormal nocturnal penile tumescence.
E. The risk of erectile dysfunction is three times greater in diabetic patients than in the general population.

**The correct response is option C.**

Sexual dysfunction in diabetic men is not limited to erectile dysfunction; it also includes ejaculatory disturbances, loss of sexual interest, persistent morning erections, and spontaneous erections.
   Erectile dysfunction in diabetic men correlates with smoking, obesity, and high levels of glycosylated hemoglobin. **(p. 363)**

17.4 Renal failure, an illness commonly encountered in psychosomatic medicine practice, often affects sexual function. Which of the following statements is *true*?

A. Entry into long-term dialysis usually alleviates sexual dysfunction.
B. The prevalence of sexual dysfunction decreases following renal transplantation for both male and female patients.
C. In men, the impact of renal failure on sexual function is "central."
D. In women, the impact of renal failure on sexual function is "gonadal."
E. Erythropoietin in men with renal failure increases gonadotropic hormone levels but does not improve sexual function.

**The correct response is option B.**

The prevalence of sexual dysfunction declines after renal transplantation.
   Entry into long-term dialysis does not appear to alleviate sexual dysfunction. In men, the impact of renal failure appears to be expressed primarily at the gonadal level. In women, the impact appears to be more marked in the central nervous system. Erythropoietin treatment of anemia in patients with renal failure both increases gonadotropic hormone levels and improves sexual function. **(p. 364)**

17.5 Psychotropic medications are commonly associated with decreased sexual function. This effect may be especially important in the medically ill. All of the following dosing strategies may be considered for selective serotonin reuptake inhibitor (SSRI)–induced sexual dysfunction *except*

A. Decreased dosage of the SSRI.
B. Change in timing of dose to several hours distant from anticipated sexual activity.
C. Drug holiday for clinically stable patient on a long-half-life SSRI.
D. Adjunctive bupropion.
E. Sildenafil.

**The correct response is option C.**

Drug holidays can be considered for patients in stable remission from depression who are taking short-half-life SSRIs (e.g., paroxetine, fluvoxamine, sertraline). **(p. 374)**

17.6 The treatment of paraphilic disorders may involve the creative application of pharmacology. All of the following statements are true *except*

  A.  Pure antiandrogens (e.g., flutamide) are usually adequate monotherapy for paraphilias.
  B.  Medroxyprogesterone acetate (MPA) inhibits androgen biosynthesis and inhibits peripheral androgen action.
  C.  MPA has a "central" effect in decreasing paraphilic fantasy.
  D.  MPA is associated with weight gain, increased systolic blood pressure, and gallstones.
  E.  Leuprolide causes a transient increase in, followed by a profound suppression of, testosterone levels.

**The correct response is option A.**

Pure antiandrogens are not adequate as monotherapy for paraphilias.

MPA is associated with weight gain, increased systolic blood pressure, gallstone formation, infertility, and possible changes in glucose tolerance. **(pp. 377–378)**

# C H A P T E R   1 8

# Substance-Related Disorders

*Select the single best response for each question.*

18.1   Which of the following definitions or statements is *false?*

A.   Physical dependence is a state of adaptation that manifests as a specific withdrawal syndrome.

B.   Withdrawal syndromes are characterized by symptoms similar to those characteristic of use of the substance.

C.   *Tolerance* is the need for increasing amounts of a substance to obtain the desired effect.

D.   Addiction is characterized by craving and impaired control of drug use despite harm.

E.   Psychological dependence is the feeling of need for a specific substance.

**The correct response is option B.**

Withdrawal encompasses a substance-specific constellation of symptoms that may occur after cessation of or decrease in use of drugs by dependent individuals. Withdrawal syndromes manifest symptoms opposite to those characteristic of use of the substance. **(p. 388)**

18.2   In Project Match, a large randomized trial of alcohol treatment modalities and predictive pretreatment variables, investigators found that the best potential predictor of a treatment outcome was

A.   Social status of the patient.

B.   Patient self-selection of treatment type.

C.   Severity of addiction.

D.   Number of previous treatment attempts.

E.   None of the above.

**The correct response is option E.**

Project Match investigators did not find a robust association between specific treatments and specific indicators (Project Match Research Group 1998). Potential predictors, such as severity of addiction, social status, number of previous treatment attempts, coping style, family history, and patient self-selection of treatment type, have not been shown to have consistent associations with treatment outcome. **(p. 391)**

18.3   Which of the following psychiatric disorders has *not* been reported to be associated with alcoholism?

A.   Bipolar disorder.

B.   Panic disorder.

C.   Social phobia.

D.   Major depressive disorder.

E.   Schizophrenia.

**The correct response is option D.**

Alcoholic patients are at increased risk of bipolar disorder, panic disorder, and social phobia but not of non-substance-induced major depressive disorder. Antisocial personality disorder also is associated with alcohol use disorders and with poorer treatment outcomes. Alcohol use is common in patients with schizophrenia, in whom such use may transiently reduce social anxiety, dysphoria, insomnia, and other nonpsychotic but unpleasant experiences. **(p. 393)**

18.4  All of the following are laboratory findings associated with alcohol abuse *except*

A.  Increased serum gamma-glutamyltransferase (SGGT) level.
B.  Decreased albumin level.
C.  Decreased serum carbohydrate-deficient transferring level.
D.  Increased uric acid level.
E.  Increased mean corpuscular volume.

**The correct response is option C.**

Serum carbohydrate-deficient transferrin is increased, not decreased, in alcohol abuse patients. Other typical findings are increased SGGT level (particularly sensitive); decreased albumin, vitamin $B_{12}$, and folic acid levels; increased uric acid and amylase levels, evidence of bone marrow suppression; increased mean corpuscular volume; increased aspartate transaminase, alanine transaminase, and lactate dehydrogenase levels; and prolonged prothrombin time (cirrhosis). **(p. 397, Table 18–4)**

18.5  Buprenorphine is

A.  A Schedule IV narcotic.
B.  An opioid agonist at higher doses.
C.  A short-acting opioid receptor antagonist.
D.  A mu opioid receptor partial agonist.
E.  None of the above.

**The correct response is option D.**

Buprenorphine, a long-acting mu opioid receptor partial agonist, was approved by the U.S. Food and Drug Administration in 2003 as a Schedule III narcotic for the treatment of opioid dependence. At lower doses, buprenorphine functions as an opioid agonist, but at higher doses it has antagonist properties. **(p. 403)**

18.6  All of the following are physical signs of phencyclidine (PCP) use *except*

A.  Nystagmus.
B.  Ataxia.
C.  Pinpoint pupils at higher doses.
D.  Hypertension.
E.  Muscle rigidity.

**The correct response is option C.**

At higher doses of PCP, dilated pupils, hypersalivation, hyperthermia, involuntary movements, and coma can occur.
    Associated physical signs include hypertension, muscle rigidity, ataxia, and nystagmus. **(p. 407)**

# Reference

Project Match Research Group: Matching alcoholism treatments to client heterogeneity: treatment main effects and matching effects on drinking during treatment. J Stud Alcohol 59:631–639, 1998

# C H A P T E R   1 9

# Heart Disease

*Select the single best response for each question.*

19.1    Depression and anxiety in heart disease patients may significantly affect quality of life and may complicate medical management. All of the following statements are true *except*

   A.  Depression is the most common comorbid psychiatric illness in coronary artery disease patients.
   B.  The prevalence of major depression following coronary artery bypass graft (CABG) is 20%–30%.
   C.  The prevalence of major depression in congestive heart failure (CHF) is 20%–30%.
   D.  Panic disorder occurs at a much higher rate in patients with mitral valve prolapse confirmed by echocardiography than in healthy control subjects.
   E.  Subsyndromal posttraumatic stress disorder (PTSD) is common in patients with automatic implantable cardioverter-defibrillators (AICDs).

**The correct response is option D.**

Panic disorder does not occur at higher-than-expected rates in patients with echocardiographically confirmed.

   Depression in coronary artery disease patients is in the 15%–20% range. Studies of depression following CABG demonstrate a prevalence of 20%–30%. Other studies have estimated a prevalence of significant depressive symptoms in 20%–30% of CHF patients. **(pp. 424–425)**

19.2    A cardiac patient presents to a psychiatrist with a complaint of mood symptoms and of seeing yellow rings around objects in the visual field. The medication most likely responsible for these symptoms is

   A.  Reserpine.
   B.  Digoxin.
   C.  Clonidine.
   D.  Beta-blocker.
   E.  Alpha-blocker.

**The correct response is option B.**

Common side effects of digoxin include visual hallucinations (classically, yellow rings around objects), delirium, and depression. **(p. 426, Table 19–1)**

19.3    Regarding psychiatric aspects of cardiovascular disease risk, all of the following are true *except*

   A.  The mortality rate for depressed coronary artery disease patients is three to four times higher than that for nondepressed coronary patients.
   B.  Depression after CABG predicts an increased risk of recurrent cardiac events within the next year.

C. Depression is associated with worsened health status in patients with coronary artery disease, whereas decreased left ventricular ejection fraction is not.
D. In depression, heightened sympathetic activity and reduced vagal tone increase the propensity for arrhythmia.
E. The SADHART study demonstrated a statistically significant positive effect of decreased cardiovascular mortality with paroxetine.

**The correct response is option E.**

In the Sertraline Antidepressant Heart Attack Trial (SADHART), sertraline, not paroxetine, demonstrated positive effects in decreased cardiovascular mortality (Glassman et al. 2002). **(p. 426, Table 19–1; pp. 427–428)**

19.4 Regarding cardiac transplantation surgery for end-stage cardiac disease and its psychiatric implications, all of the following are true *except*

A. Patients awaiting transplantation commonly experience depression secondary to their helplessness to influence their own chances of survival.
B. Patients on transplant waiting lists often experience guilt about the need for another patient to die to give them a heart.
C. Patients on transplant waiting lists tend to minimize and/or deny their illness and to display ambivalence about the surgery.
D. Patients awaiting transplant surgery are usually more anxious about the operation itself than about being excluded as a candidate.
E. Steroid-induced mood disorder and other types of depression are seen in 20%–40% of patients during the first postoperative year.

**The correct response is option D.**

Although patients awaiting transplantation are anxious about the operation, they are even more anxious about being excluded from candidacy. **(pp. 432–433)**

19.5 Regarding cardiac implications of antidepressants and antipsychotics, all of the following are true *except*

A. Tricyclic antidepressants (TCAs) can increase mortality in post–myocardial infarction (MI) patients with premature ventricular contractions (PVCs).
B. Selective serotonin reuptake inhibitors (SSRIs) plus concurrent use of beta-blockers have been shown to lead to symptomatic bradycardia.
C. Ziprasidone increases the QTc interval and has been associated with an increased risk of sudden death.
D. A QTc interval greater than 500 msec contraindicates the use of haloperidol and thioridazine.
E. Among the antipsychotics, thioridazine carries the highest risk of torsade de pointes.

**The correct response is option C.**

Ziprasidone increases the QTc interval but has not been associated with sudden death.
TCAs have quinidine-like effects on cardiac conduction and can increase mortality in post-MI patients with PVCs. Occasional cases of symptomatic bradycardia have been associated with concurrent use of SSRIs with beta-blockers. A QTc interval greater than 500 msec is considered a contraindication for haloperidol and thioridazine. Thioridazine is the antipsychotic most strongly associated with torsade de pointes. **(pp. 435–437)**

19.6   Which of the following psychotropic medications is associated with a quinidine-like type IA antiarrhythmic effect?

A. Carbamazepine.
B. Valproate.
C. Lithium carbonate.
D. Lamotrigine.
E. Buspirone.

**The correct response is option A.**

Carbamazepine resembles the TCAs in having a quinidine-like type IA antiarrhythmic effect and may cause atrioventricular conduction disturbances. **(p. 438)**

# Reference

Glassman AH, O'Connor CM, Califf RM, et al: Sertraline treatment of major depression in patients with acute MI or unstable angina. JAMA 288:701–709, 2002

# CHAPTER 20

# Lung Disease

*Select the single best response for each question.*

20.1    Which of the following statements concerning psychological factors in asthma is *false*?

   A.  People with Cluster B personality disorders are more likely to have asthma.
   B.  Brittle asthma patients are more likely to have anxiety disorders than are other asthma patients.
   C.  Anxiety and depression are associated with more respiratory symptom complaints in asthma patients.
   D.  Patients with asthma are more likely to hold catastrophic beliefs or cognitions.
   E.  Asthma attacks may be provoked by psychological distress.

**The correct response is option A.**

No particular personality type is more susceptible to the development of asthma.

Brittle asthma patients, like brittle diabetic patients, are more likely than other asthma patients to have current or past psychiatric disorders, particularly anxiety disorders, but which comes first has not been established (Garden and Ayres 1993). Anxiety and depression are associated with more respiratory symptom complaints in asthma patients but no differences in objective measures of respiratory function (Janson et al. 1994; Rietveld et al. 1999). Similar to patients with panic disorder, patients with asthma have a tendency to hold catastrophic beliefs. Asthma attacks have long been thought to be provoked by psychological distress. **(p. 446)**

20.2    In patients with chronic obstructive pulmonary disease (COPD), anxiety and depression have been found to be associated with

   A.  Higher relapse after emergency treatment.
   B.  Increased disability.
   C.  Lower exercise tolerance.
   D.  Noncompliance with treatment.
   E.  All of the above.

**The correct response is option E.**

Depression and anxiety in COPD patients have led to lower exercise tolerance (Withers et al. 1999), noncompliance with treatment (Bosley et al. 1996), and increased disability (Aydin and Ulusahin 2001). Psychological factors may predict whether a patient with COPD is at higher risk of relapse after emergency treatment. In one study, COPD patients with anxiety or depression had a higher rate of relapse within 1 month (53%) compared with those in the group without anxiety or depression (19%) (Dahlen and Janson 2002). **(p. 449)**

20.3 Regarding sarcoidosis, which of the following statements is *true*?

A. Sarcoidosis affects white patients more than African American patients.
B. In Europe, Italians have high prevalence rates.
C. Onset of the illness usually occurs between the ages of 20 and 40 years.
D. The disease follows a progressive, downhill course, with nearly 25% of patients dying from it.
E. All of the above.

**The correct response is option C.**

Onset of sarcoidosis is usually between the ages of 20 and 40 years.

Sarcoidosis affects black patients more than white patients in the United States (40 per 100,000 vs. 5 per 100,000). In Europe, Swedes and Danes have high prevalence rates. Diagnosis may be delayed by failure to recognize the slowly progressive symptoms until characteristic findings are detected on a chest X ray. The disease often follows a relapsing and remitting course, with recovery in 80% of patients, but about 5% die from sarcoidosis. **(p. 450)**


20.4 Absolute contraindications to lung transplantation include all of the following *except*

A. Alcoholism.
B. Anxiety disorders.
C. Noncompliance with treatment.
D. Hepatitis B virus.
E. Cancer.

**The correct response is option B.**

Anxiety is not an absolute contraindication to lung transplantation.

Psychiatric factors considered to be absolute contraindications include active alcoholism, drug abuse or cigarette use, severe psychiatric illness, and noncompliance with treatment (Aris et al. 1997; Paradowski 1997; Snell et al. 1993). **(p. 454)**


20.5 Theophylline has been found to reduce the effects or blood levels of which of the following psychotropic medications?

A. Lithium.
B. Fluvoxamine.
C. Carbamazepine.
D. A and C.
E. A, B, and C.

**The correct response is option D.**

Most pulmonary medications do not affect lithium levels. The exception is theophylline, which can lower lithium levels by 20%–30% and reduce the levels of carbamazepine.

Fluvoxamine tends to increase levels of theophylline. **(p. 458)**

# References

Aris RM, Gilligan PH, Neuring IP, et al: The effect of panresistant bacteria in cystic fibrosis patients on lung transplant outcome. Am J Respir Crit Care Med 155:1699–1704, 1997

Aydin IO, Ulusahin A: Depression, anxiety comorbidity, and disability in tuberculosis and chronic obstructive pulmonary disease patients: applicability of GHQ-12. Gen Hosp Psychiatry 23:77–83, 2001

Bosley CM, Corden ZM, Rees PJ, et al: Psychological factors associated with use of home nebulized therapy for COPD. Eur Respir J 9:2346–2350, 1996

Dahlen I, Janson C: Anxiety and depression are related to the outcome of emergency treatment in patients with obstructive pulmonary disease. Chest 122:1633–1637, 2002

Garden GM, Ayres JG: Psychiatric and social aspects of brittle asthma. Thorax 48:501–505, 1993

Janson C, Bjornsson E, Hetta J, et al: Anxiety and depression in relation to respiratory symptoms and asthma. Am J Respir Crit Care Med 149 (4 pt 1):930–934, 1994

Paradowski LJ: Saprophytic fungal infections and lung transplantation revisited. J Heart Lung Transplant 16:524–531, 1997

Rietveld S, van Beest I, Everaerd W: Stress-induced breathlessness in asthma. Psychol Med 29:1359–1366, 1999

Snell G, deHoyos A, Krajden M, et al: *Pseudomonas capacia* in lung transplantation recipients with cystic fibrosis. Chest 103:466–471, 1993

Withers NJ, Rudkin ST, White RJ: Anxiety and depression in severe chronic obstructive pulmonary disease: the effects of pulmonary rehabilitation. J Cardiopulm Rehabil 19:362–365, 1999

# CHAPTER 21

# Gastrointestinal Disorders

*Select the single best response for each question.*

21.1 Peptic ulcer disease is a common gastrointestinal illness, with a substantial psychiatric component in many cases. All of the following statements are true *except*

  A. The clinical use of nonsteroidal anti-inflammatory drugs (NSAIDs) has been associated with an increased risk of peptic ulcer disease.
  B. The presence of gut infection with *Helicobacter pylori* is associated with the development of peptic ulcer disease.
  C. The incidence of peptic ulcer disease has continued to increase since the 1960s.
  D. A large-scale, population-based study (Goodwin and Stein 2002) found an increased risk of generalized anxiety disorder in peptic ulcer disease patients.
  E. Psychological stress (as evidenced by anxiolytic use) is associated with peptic ulcer disease.

**The correct response is option C.**

Since the late 1960s, the overall incidence of peptic ulcer disease has begun to decline, as a result of declining rates of infection with *H. pylori*.

  *H. pylori* infection and use of NSAIDs are major risk factors for peptic ulcer disease. Smoking and psychological stress (as reflected by anxiolytic use) have also been associated with peptic ulcer disease (Anda et al. 1992; Levenstein et al. 1997; Rosenstock et al. 2003). **(pp. 466–467)**

21.2 Inflammatory bowel disease (IBD), which includes Crohn's disease and ulcerative colitis, is commonly associated with behavioral and emotional factors, which may lead to involvement of the psychosomatic medicine physician. Which of the following statements is *true*?

  A. Pathologically, ulcerative colitis is transmural, involving the full thickness of the gut.
  B. Ocular involvement in ulcerative colitis is restricted to a retinitis.
  C. The incidence of both Crohn's disease and ulcerative colitis has increased more than fivefold in the United States in the past 50 years.
  D. Because of the seriousness of medical complications, IBD patients have a higher risk of comorbid psychiatric illness compared with irritable bowel syndrome (IBS) patients.
  E. Among IBD patients, mood disorders are more common in older patients and in those with a history of previously diagnosed psychiatric illness.

**The correct response is option E.**

Among IBD patients, mood disorders are more common in older patients and in those with a previous history of psychiatric disorders.

  Ulcerative colitis is *not* transmural, and it tends to involve only the mucosa. Ulcerative colitis can produce inflammation of the skin, eyes, and joints. Whereas the incidence of Crohn's disease has increased sixfold in the past 50 years, the incidence of ulcerative colitis has remained reasonably stable. Patients with IBD show a higher prevalence of psychological disorder than the general population but a lower prevalence than patients with IBS. **(pp. 468–469)**

21.3 Irritable bowel syndrome (IBS) and functional dyspepsia are considered to be functional gastrointestinal disorders. Which of the following statements is *true*?

A. The most common functional gastrointestinal disorder is functional dyspepsia.

B. The prevalence of anxiety and mood disorders in patients with functional gastrointestinal illness is between 30% and 40%.

C. Patients with chronic functional gastrointestinal disorders are more likely to present with anxiety, whereas first-time clinic patients usually present with depression.

D. Psychiatric treatment of anxiety and mood disorders in these patients is associated with improved health-related quality of life.

E. Patients with functional dyspepsia or IBS who consult physicians are less likely to have depression than equivalent patients who do not seek medical care.

**The correct response is option D.**

Psychiatric treatment of anxiety and depression has been demonstrated to improve health-related quality of life.

The most common functional gastrointestinal disorder is IBS. The prevalence of anxiety and mood disorders in patients with functional gastrointestinal disorders is between 50% and 60%. Anxiety is more prominent in first-time clinic attenders, whereas depression seems more prominent in those who have chronic symptoms. Compared with nonconsulting patients, functional dyspepsia and IBS patients who consult physicians have more anxiety and depression and more worries about their health, especially fears of cancer. **(pp. 469–472)**

21.4 Speech therapy has been found to be useful for symptomatic relief of which of the following functional gastrointestinal illnesses?

A. Globus.

B. Gastroesophageal reflux.

C. Functional abdominal pain.

D. Cyclic vomiting.

E. IBS.

**The correct response is option A.**

Speech therapy may be helpful for globus. **(p. 472)**

21.5 Chronic hepatitis C virus (HCV) infection is a common gastrointestinal illness that often requires comprehensive multidisciplinary care. Which of the following statements is *not* true?

A. Chronic HCV infection is the major cause of chronic liver disease in the United States.

B. Major depression, posttraumatic stress disorder (PTSD), and other anxiety disorders are significantly more common in HCV patients than in control subjects.

C. HCV patients with end-stage liver disease (ESLD) have rates of depression similar to those of other ESLD patients (e.g., those with hepatitis B and alcohol-induced cirrhosis).

D. Depression is more common in HCV patients awaiting liver transplantation than in other patients awaiting transplantation.

E. Hepatitis B infection is less likely to be associated with depression than is HCV infection.

**The correct response is option C.**

Individuals with HCV infection are more likely to be depressed than are people with other forms of end-stage liver disease.

Chronic HCV, the major cause of chronic liver disease in the United States, has a prevalence of 1.8% in the population. Major depression, PTSD, and anxiety disorders, as well as alcohol- and drug-use disorders, are more prevalent in HCV patients than in control subjects. **(p. 473)**

21.6    Antidepressant therapy may be helpful in managing IBS patients. Among the following classes, which has been clearly shown to be of benefit in IBS?

   A.  Tricyclic antidepressants (TCAs).
   B.  Monoamine oxidase inhibitors (MAOIs).
   C.  Selective serotonin reuptake inhibitors (SSRIs).
   D.  Selective norepinephrine reuptake inhibitors (SNRIs).
   E.  Trazodone and nefazodone.

**The correct response is option A.**

There is clear evidence of the effectiveness of TCAs, which are effective in low doses with rapid onset. SSRIs are active at higher doses and have a slower onset of action. **(p. 475)**

# References

Anda RF, Williamson DF, Escobedo LG, et al: Self-perceived stress and the risk of peptic ulcer disease: a longitudinal study of US adults. Arch Intern Med 152:829–833, 1992

Goodwin RD, Stein MB: Generalized anxiety disorder and peptic ulcer disease among adults in the United States. Psychosom Med 64:862–866, 2002

Levenstein S, Kaplan GA, Smith MW: Psychological predictors of peptic ulcer incidence in the Alameda County Study. J Clin Gastroenterol 24:140–146, 1997

Rosenstock S, Jorgensen T, Bonnevie O, et al: Risk factors for peptic ulcer disease: a population based prospective cohort study comprising 2416 Danish adults. Gut 52:186–193, 2003

# CHAPTER 22

# Renal Disease

*Select the single best response for each question.*

22.1 Regarding end-stage renal disease (ESRD) in the United States, which of the following statements is *true*?

A. Each year nearly 80,000 Americans develop ESRD.
B. In 2001, more than 290,000 patients were receiving dialysis in the United States.
C. Nearly 8 million individuals are estimated to have chronic renal insufficiency.
D. A and C.
E. A, B, and C.

**The correct response is option E.**

Each year, approximately 80,000 Americans develop ESRD. In 2001, the dialysis population numbered 292,215 patients (U.S. Renal Data System 2003). An additional 8 million individuals are estimated to have chronic renal insufficiency (Robertson et al. 2002). **(p. 483)**

22.2 In a review of psychiatric illness involving 200,000 U.S. dialysis patients, it was reported that

A. Nearly 10% had been hospitalized with a psychiatric diagnosis.
B. Dementia was the most common psychiatric illness.
C. Compared with other medical illnesses, the primary diagnosis of depression was higher in patients with ischemic heart disease than in patients with renal failure.
D. A and C.
E. A, B, and C.

**The correct response is option A.**

Among these dialysis patients, almost 10% had previously been hospitalized with a psychiatric diagnosis, and for 25% of this subgroup the psychiatric diagnosis was the primary reason for hospitalization (Kimmel et al. 1993).

Depression and other affective disorders were the most common diagnoses, followed by delirium and dementia. The primary diagnosis of depression was more frequent in renal failure patients than in those with ischemic heart disease or cerebrovascular disease (Kimmel et al. 1993). **(p. 484)**

22.3 Dialysis encephalopathy, a serious cognitive disorder seen in dialysis patients in the 1970s and 1980s, was believed to be caused by

A. Azotemia.
B. Aluminum found in phosphate-binding gels.
C. Metabolic acidosis.
D. Hyperkalemia.
E. Hyperphosphatemia.

**The correct response is option B.**

"Dialysis encephalopathy" or "dialysis dementia" was the most serious cognitive disorder seen in dialysis patients in the 1970s and 1980s. This usually fatal syndrome occurred in patients who had been on hemodialysis for at least 2 years; early signs included memory impairment, dysarthria, stuttering speech, depression, and psychosis. Aluminum was considered the most likely culprit, and it was found in phosphate-binding gels and in trace amounts in dialysate water.

Metabolic abnormalities such as hyperkalemia, hyperphosphatemia, metabolic acidosis, and azotemia (elevated blood urea nitrogen [BUN] and creatinine levels) are seen in end-stage renal disease. **(pp. 485–486)**

22.4 According to recently published U.S. guidelines (Moss et al. 2000), which of the following conditions is *not* an appropriate reason to withhold dialysis?

A. End-stage cancer.
B. Permanent unconsciousness (as in a persistent vegetative state).
C. Severe delirium.
D. Severe, continued, and unrelenting pain.
E. Multiple organ system failure in a hospitalized patient.

**The correct response is option C.**

Severe delirium is *not* an appropriate reason to withhold dialysis. Valid rationales for withholding dialysis include severe/irreversible dementia, permanent unconsciousness, severe/continued/unrelenting pain, and multiple organ system failure. **(p. 488)**

22.5 Which of the following forms of psychotherapy has been shown to be helpful in treating patients with end-stage renal disease?

A. Cognitive-behavioral therapy (CBT).
B. Hypnosis.
C. Behavioral interventions.
D. Group therapy.
E. All of the above.

**The correct response is option E.**

In a recent study of Japanese hemodialysis patients (Sagawa et al. 2003), CBT achieved a 65% reduction of fluid intake. In a study of five Boston patients (Surman and Tolkoff-Rubin 1984), hypnosis was successful in curtailing psychiatric symptoms. In a study of 116 patients, Cummings et al. (1981) demonstrated that behavioral contracting and weekly telephone contacts were effective in the short term in improving compliance with medical regimens. A controlled trial of group therapy in Israeli dialysis patients showed a significant decrease in psychological distress and interdialytic weight gain in those who received group therapy (Auslander and Buchs 2002). Any form of psychotherapy stands the best chance of success if conducted during dialysis treatment sessions (Levy 1999). **(p. 489)**

# References

Auslander GK, Buchs A: Evaluating an activity intervention with hemodialysis patients in Israel. Soc Work Health Care 35:407–423, 2002

Cummings KB, Becker M, Kirscht JP, et al: Intervention strategies to improve compliance with medical regimens by ambulatory hemodialysis patients. J Behav Med 4:111–127, 1981

Kimmel PL, Weihs K, Peterson RA: Survival in hemodialysis patients: the role of depression. J Am Soc Nephrol 3:12–27, 1993

Levy NB: Renal failure, dialysis and transplantation, in Psychiatric Treatment of the Medically Ill. Edited by Robinson RG. New York, Marcel Dekker, 1999, pp 141–153

Moss AH, Renal Physicians Association, American Society of Nephrology Working Group: a new clinical practice guideline on initiation and withdrawal of dialysis that makes explicit the role of palliative medicine. J Palliat Med 3:253–260, 2000

Robertson S, Newbigging K, Isles CG, et al: High incidence of renal failure requiring short-term dialysis: a prospective observational study. Q J Med 95:585–590, 2002

Sagawa M, Oka M, Chaboyer W: The utility of cognitive behavioural therapy on chronic haemodialysis patients' fluid intake: a preliminary examination. Int J Nurs Stud 40:367–373, 2003

Surman OS, Tolkoff-Rubin N: Use of hypnosis in patients receiving hemodialysis for end stage renal disease. Gen Hosp Psychiatry 6:31–35, 1984

U.S. Renal Data System: Excerpts from the USRDS 2002 Annual Data Report: Atlas of End-Stage Renal Disease in the United States. Am J Kidney Dis 41 (suppl 2):S15–S28, S135–S150, 2003

# C H A P T E R   2 3

# Endocrine and Metabolic Disorders

*Select the single best response for each question.*

23.1   The psychiatric care of diabetes mellitus (DM) poses several challenges for both psychiatric illness management and patients' global levels of health and functioning. Specifically, mood disorders are a significant problem in this population. All of the following are true *except*

    A.   Psychiatric disorders are associated with treatment noncompliance and vascular complications in type 1, but not type 2, diabetes.

    B.   The prevalence of depression in diabetic patients is two to three times higher than that in the general population.

    C.   Lustman et al. (2000) have postulated that depression and poor glycemic control are reciprocally linked.

    D.   Depression in diabetes mellitus typically antedates the development of vascular complications.

    E.   Conventional treatments for mood disorders in diabetes mellitus lead to improved glycemic control as well as improvement in depression symptoms.

**The correct response is option A.**

In both type 1 and type 2 diabetes, psychiatric disorders are associated with treatment noncompliance and vascular complications.

    Depression typically occurs early in diabetes mellitus, before the appearance of vascular complications (Jacobson et al. 2002; Kovacs et al. 1997; Mayou et al. 1991). The prevalence of depression in diabetes mellitus is two to three times higher than that in the general population. Treatment of depression in diabetes mellitus can lead to improved treatment adherence and improved glycemic control. **(pp. 496–498)**

23.2   Besides depressive disorders, other psychiatric illnesses are of clinical importance in diabetes. Which of the following statements is *true*?

    A.   The high risk of diabetes in bipolar disorder patients primarily relates to type 1 diabetes.

    B.   In bipolar disorder patients with type 2 diabetes, any excess weight is accounted for by weight gain from psychotropic medications.

    C.   The risk of type 2 diabetes in schizophrenia is approximately 1.5 times that in the general population.

    D.   It is believed that antagonism of 5-HT$_{1A}$ receptors may lead to decreased levels of insulin and increased blood glucose in schizophrenic patients treated with atypical antipsychotics.

    E.   The increased risk of diabetes in schizophrenia is primarily due to the use of atypical antipsychotics.

**The correct response is option D.**

Antagonism of 5-HT$_{1A}$ receptors may play a role in decreasing levels of insulin and increasing hyperglycemia.

The high risk of diabetes in bipolar patients is associated with but not fully accounted for by weight gain–associated psychotropic drugs. The risk of developing type 2 diabetes is two to four times greater in patients with schizophrenia than in the general population. The increased risk of diabetes in schizophrenia precedes the use of atypical agents. **(pp. 498–499)**

23.3    Diabetes has been associated with effects on cognitive function. Which of the following statements is *not* true?

A. The onset of diabetes before age 6 years is associated with cognitive impairment.
B. In longitudinal studies of pediatric diabetes patients tested at 2 and 6 years after diagnosis (Northam et al. 1998), speed of information processing, vocabulary, and block design performance were worse in patients than in control subjects.
C. Recurrent episodes of hypoglycemia are associated with poorer learning and short-term memory performance.
D. Chronic hyperglycemia is associated with poorer visual organization skills.
E. The significantly increased risk for dementia in diabetes is due to the heightened risks both for Alzheimer's dementia and for vascular dementia.

**The correct response is option E.**

Two studies showed a 60%–100% increased risk for cognitive decline among patients with diabetes as compared with those without diabetes (Gregg and Brown 2003). This increased risk appears to be mediated primarily by an increase in vascular dementia rather than a heightened risk for Alzheimer's disease. **(pp. 499–500)**

23.4    Hyperthyroidism is a useful clinical model for psychiatric illness arising from metabolic disturbance. The symptoms of hyperthyroidism converge with those of several psychiatric illness groups. All of the following are true *except*

A. Presence and severity of psychiatric symptoms in Graves' disease correlate directly with thyroid hormone levels.
B. Graves' disease is associated with anxiety, depression, hypomania, and cognitive impairment.
C. According to Stern et al. (1996), the most common symptoms self-reported by hyperthyroidism patients were irritability, shakiness, and anxiety.
D. Anti-thyroid therapy is associated with improvement in depression symptoms.
E. Hyperthyroidism with anxious dysphoria is more common in younger, rather than older, patients.

**The correct response is option A.**

Physiological and psychiatric symptoms correlated poorly with thyroid hormone levels in Graves' disease patients (Trzepacz et al. 1989).

Graves' disease is associated with anxiety, hypomania, depression, and cognitive difficulties, which may improve with anti-thyroid treatment. Anxious dysphoria is more common in younger patients. **(pp. 500–501)**

23.5 Hypothyroidism offers another model of an endocrinologically based psychiatric illness. Regarding hypothyroidism and psychiatric illness, which of the following statements is *true*?

A. An elevated serum thyroid-stimulating hormone (TSH) concentration serves both to screen for and to confirm hypothyroidism.
B. Grade 1 hypothyroidism involves overt clinical symptoms, elevated TSH, and low serum thyroxine ($T_4$) concentrations.
C. Subclinical hypothyroidism is equally common in men and women.
D. Cognitive impairment in hypothyroidism may be independent of mood disturbance.
E. Subclinical hypothyroidism is most common in bipolar patients with euphoric mania without rapid mood cycling.

The correct response is option D.

In some cases of hypothyroidism, cognitive problems are independent of depression. Burmeister et al. (2001) found no relationship between cognitive ability and level of depression in a group of hypothyroid patients. (pp. 501–502)

23.6 Adrenal cortical disease may readily come to the attention of the psychosomatic medicine physician. Notably, depression is commonly reported in Cushing's syndrome of excessive adrenocorticotropic hormone (ACTH). Which of the following depression-spectrum symptoms is *not* characteristic of a typical case of depression associated with Cushing's syndrome?

A. Hypersomnia.
B. Irritable mood.
C. Crying.
D. Decreased energy.
E. Suicidal ideation.

The correct response is option A.

Hypersomnia is not characteristically found in Cushing's syndrome patients. Depression is the most prevalent psychiatric disturbance, accompanied by irritability, insomnia, crying, decreased energy and libido, poor concentration and memory, and suicidal ideation. (p. 503)

23.7 Various antipsychotic agents are associated with increased serum prolactin and resultant systemic complications. Which of the following atypical antipsychotic agents carries the highest risk of increased prolactin?

A. Clozapine.
B. Olanzapine.
C. Ziprasidone.
D. Risperidone.
E. Quetiapine.

The correct response is option D.

Risperidone raises the serum prolactin concentration by an average of 45–80 ng/mL, with larger increases in women than in men.

   Clozapine, quetiapine, and olanzapine either cause no increase in prolactin secretion or increase prolactin transiently. (p. 506)

# References

Burmeister LA, Ganguli M, Dodge HH, et al: Hypothyroidism and cognition: preliminary evidence for a specific defect in memory. Thyroid 11:1177–1185, 2001

Gregg E, Brown A: Cognitive and physical disabilities and aging-related complications of diabetes. Clinical Diabetes 21:113–116, 2003

Jacobson AM, Samson JA, Weinger K, et al: Diabetes, the brain, and behavior: is there a biological mechanism underlying the association between diabetes and depression? Int Rev Neurobiol 51:455–479, 2002

Kovacs M, Obrosky DS, Goldston D, et al: Major depressive disorder in youths with IDDM: a controlled prospective study of course and outcome. Diabetes Care 20:45–51, 1997

Lustman PJ, Anderson RJ, Freedland KE, et al: Depression and poor glycemic control: a meta-analytic review of the literature. Diabetes Care 23:934–942, 2000

Mayou R, Peveler R, Davies B, et al: Psychiatric morbidity in young adults with insulin-dependent diabetes mellitus. Psychol Med 21:639–645, 1991

Northam EA, Anderson PJ, Werther GA, et al: Neuropsychological complications of IDDM in children 2 years after disease onset. Diabetes Care 21:379–384, 1998

Stern RA, Robinson B, Thorner AR, et al: A survey study of neuropsychiatric complaints in patients with Graves' disease. J Neuropsychiatry Clin Neurosci 8:181, 1996

Trzepacz PT, Klein I, Roberts M, et al: Graves' disease: an analysis of thyroid hormone levels and hyperthyroid signs and symptoms. Am J Med 87:558–561, 1989

# C H A P T E R   2 4

# Oncology

*Select the single best response for each question.*

24.1    Many research groups have assessed depression in cancer patients. Cancer types highly associated with depression include all of the following *except*

    A. Breast cancer.
    B. Lymphoma.
    C. Lung cancer.
    D. Oropharyngeal cancer.
    E. Pancreatic cancer.

**The correct response is option B.**

Cancer types highly associated with depression include oropharyngeal (22%–57%), pancreatic (33%–50%), breast (1.5%–46%), and lung (11%–44%). The prevalence of depression is reported to be less in patients with other cancers, such as colon cancer (13%–25%), gynecological cancer (12%–23%), and lymphoma (8%–19%) (Massie 2004). **(p. 518)**

24.2    An increased risk of suicide in cancer patients is associated with all of the following *except*

    A. Advanced stage of disease.
    B. Inadequately controlled pain.
    C. Social isolation.
    D. Female gender.
    E. History of psychiatric illness.

**The correct response is option D.**

An increased risk of suicide in cancer patients is associated with male gender, advanced stage of disease, poor prognosis, delirium with poor impulse control, inadequately controlled pain, depression, history of psychiatric illness, current or previous alcohol or substance abuse, previous suicide attempts, physical and emotional exhaustion, social isolation, and extreme need for control. Recognition of suicidal thoughts should lead to emergent psychiatric evaluation with frank discussion. **(p. 519)**

24.3    Common causes of cancer-related fatigue include which of the following cancer treatments?

    A. Interferon.
    B. Chemotherapy.
    C. Irradiation.
    D. All of the above.
    E. None of the above.

**The correct response is option D.**

Cancer-related fatigue is caused by interferon, chemotherapy, and radiation therapy, in addition to pain, hormonal imbalances, drug effects of opioids and sedatives, and psychiatric disorders such as depression and sleep disruption. **(p. 522, Table 24–2)**

24.4    In general, which of the following variables is associated with *less* mental distress in men with prostate cancer?

A.  More serious disease.
B.  Undergoing radiation treatment.
C.  Younger age.
D.  Undergoing surgery.
E.  None of the above.

**The correct response is option D.**

In general, men undergoing surgery, older men, and men with less serious disease have less mental distress (Litwin et al. 2002). **(p. 523)**

24.5    One of the two most significant risk factors for breast cancer is family history. What is the other significant risk factor?

A.  Increasing age.
B.  Other physical illness.
C.  Autoimmune disorder.
D.  Depression.
E.  Past psychiatric illness.

**The correct response is option A.**

The two most significant risk factors for breast cancer are increasing age and family history. **(p. 524)**

# References

Litwin MS, Lubeck DP, Spitalny GM, et al: Mental health in men treated for early stage prostate carcinoma. Cancer 95:54–60, 2002

Massie MJ: Prevalence of depression in patients with cancer. J Natl Cancer Inst Monogr 32:57–71, 2004

# C H A P T E R   2 5

# Rheumatology

*Select the single best response for each question.*

25.1 Depression is a common problem in rheumatoid arthritis. However, consideration of the specific needs and complexity of these patients is important. Which is the recommended first-line pharmacological management strategy for depression in rheumatoid arthritis?

A. Selective serotonin reuptake inhibitors (SSRIs), with doses limited to one-half the usual adult dose.
B. SSRIs, in typical adult doses.
C. Tricyclic antidepressants (TCAs), limited to low doses only.
D. TCAs in low doses, routinely combined with SSRIs.
E. Full-dose TCAs.

**The correct response is option B.**

SSRIs, such as fluoxetine or citalopram, in doses to recommended maxima should be considered as first-line treatment for depression in rheumatoid arthritis.

TCAs in low doses are useful only for pain relief. Combined use of TCAs and SSRIs greatly increases the risk of adverse events and should be avoided unless done under expert guidance. **(p. 537)**

25.2 Regarding central nervous system (CNS) or psychiatric complications in rheumatoid arthritis, which of the following statements is *not* true?

A. Neurological complications are common in rheumatoid arthritis due to direct CNS involvement.
B. Psychiatric illness in rheumatoid arthritis usually relates to emotional reactions to having a serious systemic illness.
C. Depressive symptoms correlate with levels of physical pain in rheumatoid arthritis.
D. The association between rheumatoid arthritis and psychiatric symptoms is strongest for patients with more serious disease.
E. Neuroticism in rheumatoid arthritis patients is associated with more distress, regardless of pain levels.

**The correct response is option A.**

Neurological complications in rheumatoid arthritis are *not* common, and direct involvement of the CNS is rare. **(pp. 538–540)**

25.3 Which of the following is *not* associated with greater risk of depression in osteoarthritis?

A. Older age.
B. Lower level of education.
C. Greater self-reported impact of osteoarthritis on patient's life.
D. More pain.
E. Objective measures of functional disability.

The correct response is option A.

When depression occurs in patients with osteoarthritis, it has been shown to be associated with a number of factors: younger age, less education, higher pain, and greater self-reported impact of the disease. **(p. 542)**

25.4  Systemic lupus erythematosus (SLE) is a complicated rheumatological disease known to be associated with psychiatric comorbidity. Regarding psychiatric manifestations of SLE, all of the following are true *except*

A. Neuropsychiatric manifestations in SLE have a prevalence of between 75% and 90%.
B. In SLE, the presence of antiribosomal P antibodies has been consistently associated with psychosis and severe depression.
C. Antiphospholipid antibodies (e.g., anticardiolipin) are associated with stroke and cognitive impairment.
D. SLE-associated psychosis, depression, mania, and anxiety are at least partially reversible with intervention.
E. SLE-related cognitive impairment may respond to corticosteroid treatment.

**The correct response is option B.**

Antiribosomal P antibodies have been associated with psychosis and severe depression, although not consistently.

Neuropsychiatric manifestations in SLE range from stroke, seizures, headaches, neuropathy, transverse myelitis, and movement disorders to cognitive deficits, depression, mania, anxiety, psychosis, and delirium. **(pp. 542–545)**

25.5  Among the neuropsychiatric syndromes in SLE specified by the American College of Rheumatology (1999), which of the following is the most common?

A. Mood disorders.
B. Anxiety disorders.
C. Psychosis.
D. Cognitive dysfunction.
E. Acute confusional state/delirium.

**The correct response is option D.**

Cognitive dysfunction is the most common neuropsychiatric disorder in patients with SLE, affecting up to 80% of SLE patients. Depression is the second most common disorder, present in approximately 50% of patients. It is unclear whether anxiety is attributable to direct CNS involvement or simply a reaction to chronic illness. Distinguishing psychosis caused by CNS lupus from corticosteroid-induced psychosis presents a major diagnostic challenge. Delirium is common in severe SLE. **(p. 544)**

25.6  In the management of SLE, use of high-dose corticosteroids is necessary and thus common. Corticosteroids are themselves associated with psychiatric side effects. However, psychiatric comorbidity of SLE independent of the use of corticosteroids may make the sorting out of symptoms and causal factors difficult. Which of the following statements is *not* true?

A. The reporting of severe psychiatric symptoms in SLE cases antedated the use of corticosteroids.
B. Psychiatric symptoms are more common and more severe in SLE patients receiving corticosteroids than in patients being treated with corticosteroids for other illnesses.

C. Psychiatric symptoms in SLE patients often improve with corticosteroid therapy.

D. In SLE patients, reduction or discontinuation of corticosteroids may exacerbate psychiatric symptoms.

E. SLE patients who experience psychosis during a course of corticosteroids usually will have a recurrence of psychosis with steroid retreatment.

**The correct response is option E.**

In SLE patients who have had a previous psychotic episode while taking corticosteroids, retreatment usually does not precipitate a recurrence of the psychosis. **(p. 545)**

25.7   Confusion, psychosis, mania, aggression, depression, nightmares, anxiety, aggression, and delirium have all been associated with which of the following medications for SLE?

A. Gold salts.

B. Penicillamine.

C. Azathioprine.

D. Leflunomide.

E. Hydroxychloroquine.

**The correct response is option E.**

Hydroxychloroquine produces many psychiatric side effects. Gold salts and penicillamine do not appear to produce psychiatric side effects; azathioprine may cause delirium. **(p. 549, Table 25–3)**

# Reference

American College of Rheumatology Ad Hoc Committee on Neuropsychiatric Lupus Nomenclature: Nomenclature and case definitions for neuropsychiatric lupus syndromes. Arthritis Rheum 42:599–608, 1999

# C H A P T E R   2 6

# Chronic Fatigue and Fibromyalgia Syndromes

*Select the single best response for each question.*

26.1    All of the following psychiatric disorders are among the exclusion criteria for chronic fatigue syndrome *except*

A.  Dementia.
B.  Anorexia or bulimia nervosa.
C.  Unipolar depression without melancholia.
D.  Alcohol or substance misuse.
E.  Bipolar depression.

**The correct response is option C.**

Unipolar depression without melancholia is *not* an exclusion criterion for chronic fatigue syndrome. **(p. 557)**

26.2    The American College of Rheumatology (ACR) has developed diagnostic criteria for fibromyalgia. Which of the following are included in the criteria?

A.  Widespread pain.
B.  Symptom duration of at least 1 year.
C.  Pain at 11 or more of 18 specific sites on the body.
D.  A and C.
E.  A, B, and C.

**The correct response is option D.**

The ACR criteria published in 1990 are the most widely accepted (Wolfe et al. 1990). These specify widespread pain of at least 3 months' duration and tenderness at 11 or more of 18 specific sites on the body. **(p. 557)**

26.3    Which of the following psychiatric disorders is most commonly found in patients with chronic fatigue syndrome or fibromyalgia syndrome?

A.  Depression.
B.  Psychosis.
C.  Anxiety.
D.  A and C.
E.  A, B, and C.

**The correct response is option D.**

In clinical practice, many but not all patients with chronic fatigue syndrome or fibromyalgia syndrome can be given a psychiatric diagnosis. Most will meet criteria for depression or an anxiety syndrome. **(p. 559)**

26.4    Which of the following is one of the best-supported biological abnormalities reported to be associated with both chronic fatigue syndrome and fibromyalgia syndrome?

A.  Low blood levels of cortisol.
B.  High blood levels of cortisol.
C.  Low cerebrospinal fluid (CSF) levels of substance P.
D.  Elevated blood pressure.
E.  Abnormalities of muscle metabolism.

**The correct response is option A.**

One of the best-supported biological abnormalities reported to be associated with both chronic fatigue syndrome and fibromyalgia syndrome is changes in neuroendocrine stress hormones. A repeated observation has been a tendency toward low blood levels of cortisol and a poor cortisol response to stress (Parker et al. 2001). This finding differs from what would be expected in depression (in which blood levels of cortisol are typically elevated) but is similar to effects reported in other stress-induced and anxiety states. It is not known whether these changes in neuroendocrine stress hormones represent a primary abnormality or merely a consequence of inactivity or sleep disruption, however.

Patients with fibromyalgia syndrome also show elevated cerebrospinal fluid levels of substance P (Russell et al. 1994). However, elevated substance P has not been found in chronic fatigue syndrome patients (Evengard et al. 1998). Failure to maintain blood pressure when assuming erect posture (orthostatic intolerance)—and particularly a pattern in which the heart rate increases abnormally (postural orthostatic tachycardia syndrome)—has been reported in both chronic fatigue syndrome (Rowe et al. 1995) and fibromyalgia syndrome (Bou-Holaigah et al. 1997). **(pp. 562–563)**

26.5    All of the following medical disorders are commonly found in patients with either chronic fatigue syndrome or fibromyalgia syndrome *except*

A.  Sleep apnea.
B.  Rheumatoid arthritis.
C.  Spinal stenosis.
D.  Anemia.
E.  Thyroid disorders.

**The correct response is option B.**

Rheumatoid arthritis is uncommon (~1 per 2,500–1,000,000 cases) in fibromyalgia syndrome; the incidence of sleep apnea, spinal stenosis, anemia, and thyroid disorders is approximately 1 per 100 cases. **(p. 566, Table 26–4)**

# References

Bou-Holaigah I, Calkins H, Flynn JA, et al: Provocation of hypotension and pain during upright tilt table testing in adults with fibromyalgia. Clin Exp Rheumatol 15:239–246, 1997

Evengard B, Nilsson CG, Lindh G, et al: Chronic fatigue syndrome differs from fibromyalgia: no evidence for elevated substance P levels in cerebrospinal fluid of patients with chronic fatigue syndrome. Pain 78:153–155, 1998

Parker AJ, Wessely S, Cleare AJ: The neuroendocrinology of chronic fatigue syndrome and fibromyalgia. Psychol Med 31:1331–1345, 2001

Rowe PC, Bou Holaigah I, Kan JS, et al: Is neurally mediated hypotension an unrecognised cause of chronic fatigue? Lancet 345:623–624, 1995

Russell IJ, Orr MD, Littman B, et al: Elevated cerebrospinal fluid levels of substance P in patients with the fibromyalgia syndrome. Arthritis Rheum 37:1593–1601, 1994

Wolfe F, Smythe HA, Yunus MB, et al: The American College of Rheumatology 1990 criteria for the classification of fibromyalgia: report of the Multicenter Criteria Committee. Arthritis Rheum 33:160–172, 1990

# C H A P T E R    2 7

# Infectious Diseases

*Select the single best response for each question.*

27.1 Pediatric autoimmune neuropsychiatric disorder associated with streptococcal infection (PANDAS) offers a compelling model for infectious disease–induced psychiatric illness. All of the following are true regarding PANDAS *except*

A. Seventy percent of children with Sydenham's chorea have obsessive-compulsive symptoms before the onset of chorea.
B. PANDAS consists of obsessive-compulsive and tic symptoms that occur following group A beta-hemolytic streptococcus (GABHS) infection.
C. The infection most commonly implicated is pharyngitis.
D. Antistreptolysin-O (ASO) titers rise with GABHS infections, and levels covary with symptoms.
E. Because of the high specificity of ASO titers in evaluation, throat cultures are superfluous.

**The correct response is option E.**

Because some children with GABHS infection may have a sore throat, throat cultures are recommended in addition to ASO titers. **(p. 579)**

27.2 Rocky Mountain spotted fever (RMSF) is another infectious disease that is associated with neuropsychiatric complications. Which of the following statements is *true*?

A. The responsible organism is *Rickettsia prowazekii*.
B. Central nervous system (CNS) involvement is seen in 25% of RMSF cases and includes lethargy, confusion, and delirium.
C. Irritability, personality changes, and apathy may occur before the rash in RMSF, most commonly in elderly individuals.
D. Encephalopathy in RMSF is rare unless computed tomography (CT) or magnetic resonance imaging (MRI) scans are abnormal.
E. Well over 50% of U.S. RMSF cases occur in the mountainous west.

**The correct response is option B.**

CNS involvement occurs in 25% of RMSF cases and includes lethargy, confusion, and occasionally fulminant delirium.

The responsible organism is *Rickettsia rickettsii*. Irritability, personality changes, and apathy may occur before the rash, particularly in children. Encephalopathy is seen in 80% of patients with normal scans. Half of U.S. cases occur in the South Atlantic region. **(p. 580)**

27.3 Which of the following psychiatric symptoms is *not* characteristic of classic chronic Lyme disease encephalopathy?

A. Poor concentration.
B. Amnesia.
C. Fatigue.
D. Psychosis.
E. Depression.

**The correct response is option D.**

Psychosis is not characteristic of chronic Lyme encephalopathy. Typical symptoms include difficulty with concentration and memory, fatigue, daytime hypersomnolence, irritability, and depression. **(p. 583)**

27.4 Herpes simplex virus (HSV) infection can result in encephalitis that may come to the attention of the psychosomatic medicine psychiatrist. Which of the following statements is *not* true?

A. Electroencephalogram (EEG) testing is both sensitive and specific, with findings of periodic temporal spikes and slow waves.
B. Brain biopsy has a high diagnostic yield and a low complication rate.
C. Acyclovir is the drug treatment of choice.
D. Klüver-Bucy syndrome is a possible sequela.
E. HSV encephalitis is associated with olfactory hallucinations.

**The correct response is option A.**

EEG is a sensitive but nonspecific diagnostic test for HSV encephalitis, showing periodic temporal spikes and slow waves as opposed to the more diffuse changes usually seen in other forms of viral encephalitis. **(p. 586)**

27.5 Viral hepatitis is a common clinical problem with psychiatric implications. Which of the following statements is *true*?

A. Depression is a contraindication to interferon therapy.
B. Fatigue in chronic hepatitis is more closely related to disease severity than to depression or social factors.
C. Depression is uncommon in hepatitis C and B infections.
D. Depression is induced in 20%–40% of patients treated with interferon.
E. Depression induced by interferon is not responsive to selective serotonin reuptake inhibitors (SSRIs).

**The correct response is option D.**

Treatment with interferon causes depression in 20%–40% of patients.

Depression associated with hepatitis or interferon is amenable to treatment with antidepressants; therefore, depression should *not* be considered a contraindication to interferon therapy. Dosing should be adjusted downward for patients with impaired liver function. Fatigue in chronic hepatitis is more closely correlated with depression and other psychological factors than with severity of hepatitis. Depression is frequently comorbid, especially in the chronic forms of hepatitis B and C infection. **(pp. 587–588)**

27.6    Meningoencephalitis with prominent somnolence, colloquially known as sleeping sickness, is associated with which of the following infections?

   A.  Neurocysticercosis.
   B.  Toxoplasmosis.
   C.  Trypanosomiasis.
   D.  Malaria.
   E.  Schistosomiasis.

**The correct response is option C.**

Trypanosomiasis, caused by a subspecies of *Trypanosoma brucei*, is transmitted to humans and animals by the bite of the blood-sucking tsetse fly.

   Neurocysticercosis, an infection of the CNS caused by the larval form of *Taenia solium*, is the leading cause of seizures in adults in endemic areas. Other psychiatric symptoms include depression, psychosis, and cognitive decline. Malaria, caused by *Plasmodium falciparum*, begins with disorientation, mild stupor, and psychosis and rapidly progresses to seizures and coma with decerebrate posturing. Schistosomiasis, caused by trematodes of the genus *Schistosoma*, has few CNS symptoms. **(p. 590)**

27.7    Which of the following antibiotics has been associated with psychosis, paranoia, mania, agitation, and a Tourette-like syndrome?

   A.  Cephalosporins.
   B.  Quinolones.
   C.  Trimethoprim–sulfamethoxazole.
   D.  Gentamicin.
   E.  Clarithromycin.

**The correct response is option B.**

The side effects of quinolones include psychosis, paranoia, mania, agitation, and a Tourette-like syndrome.

   Cephalosporins can cause euphoria, delusions, depersonalization, and illusions; trimethoprim–sulfamethoxazole and gentamicin, delirium and psychosis; and clarithromycin, delirium and mania. **(p. 592, Table 27–3)**

# C H A P T E R 2 8

# HIV/AIDS

*Select the single best response for each question.*

28.1 The most common neoplasm seen in AIDS patients is

A. Sarcoma.
B. Lung cancer.
C. Pancreatic cancer.
D. Colon cancer.
E. Lymphoma.

**The correct response is option E.**

Lymphoma is the most common central nervous system (CNS) neoplasm seen in AIDS patients, affecting between 0.6% and 3.0%. The patient is generally afebrile; may develop a single lesion with focal neurological signs or small, multifocal lesions; and most commonly presents with mental status change. Seizures occur in about 15% of these patients. **(p. 601)**

28.2 The addition of zidovudine to antiviral treatment regimens for HIV infection has resulted in

A. Worsening of cognitive functioning.
B. Improvement in cognitive functioning.
C. Onset of parkinsonian symptoms.
D. Increased risk for psychosis.
E. Increased delirium.

**The correct response is option B.**

Initial open-label studies of zidovudine showed promising results, with patients improving on neuropsychological tests (Fischl et al. 1987). The AIDS Clinical Trials Group trial compared high doses of zidovudine with placebo but was stopped prematurely after preliminary data showed dramatic cognitive improvement in those receiving zidovudine (Sidtis et al. 1993). A sharp decline in the incidence of HIV-associated dementia was observed following widespread use of zidovudine (Chiesi et al. 1990, 1996; Portegies et al. 1989), and HIV-associated dementia became rare in patients receiving continued zidovudine treatment (Portegies et al. 1989). Zidovudine might also produce improvement in patients already affected by dementia (Tozzi et al. 1993; Vion-Dury et al. 1995). **(p. 605)**

28.3 HIV is believed to increase the risk of developing major depression through which of the following mechanisms?

A. Chronic stress.
B. Worsening social isolation.
C. Demoralization.
D. Direct injury to subcortical brain areas.
E. All of the above.

**The correct response is option E.**

HIV increases the risk of developing major depression through a variety of mechanisms, including direct injury to subcortical areas of brain, chronic stress, worsening social isolation, and intense demoralization. Direct evidence for a relationship between worsening HIV disease and the development of major depression is limited, but several studies have supported this link, particularly the Multicenter AIDS Cohort Study (Lyketsos et al. 1996). This study showed that rates of depression increased 2.5-fold as CD4 cells declined to fewer than 200/mm³ just before patients developed AIDS, suggesting that lower CD4 cell counts predict increased rates of depression. **(p. 606)**

28.4 AIDS mania often has a clinical profile different from that of primary mania. All of the following are characteristics of AIDS mania *except*

A. Irritable mood.
B. Infrequent spontaneous remissions.
C. Psychomotor agitation.
D. More chronic than episodic.
E. None of the above.

**The correct response is option C.**

AIDS mania seems to have a clinical profile somewhat different from that of primary mania. Irritable mood is often a prominent feature, but elevated mood can be observed. Sometimes prominent psychomotor slowing accompanying the cognitive slowing of AIDS dementia will replace the expected hyperactivity of mania, which complicates the differential diagnosis. AIDS mania is usually quite severe in its presentation and malignant in its course. AIDS mania seems to be more chronic than episodic, with infrequent spontaneous remissions, and usually relapses with cessation of treatment. Because of their cognitive deficits, patients have little functional reserve to begin with and are less able to pursue treatment independently or consistently. **(p. 610)**

28.5 Which of the following personality characteristics best describes the majority of patients who would be seen in an AIDS clinic in a metropolitan area?

A. Unstable extrovert.
B. Stable extrovert.
C. Unstable introvert.
D. Stable introvert.
E. None of the above.

**The correct response is option A.**

Unstable extroverts are the most prone to engage in practices that place them at risk for HIV. In the psychiatry service of the Johns Hopkins AIDS clinic (a referral-biased sample), about 60% of patients present with this blend of extroversion and emotional instability (Lyketsos et al. 1994). Unstable extroverts are more likely to engage in behavior that places them at risk for HIV infection and are more likely to pursue sex promiscuously.

The second most common personality type is that of the stable extrovert. Introverted personalities appear to be less common. Their focus on the future, avoidance of negative consequences, and preference for cognition over feeling render them more likely to engage in protective and preventative behaviors. Unstable introverts are anxious, moody, and pessimistic. Typically, they seek drugs and/or sex not for pleasure, but for relief or distraction from pain. Stable introverts are least likely to engage in risky or hedonistic behaviors. They are HIV-positive, typically, as a result of a blood transfusion or an occupational needle stick. **(pp. 613–614)**

# References

Chiesi A, Agresti MG, Dally LG, et al: Decrease in notifications of AIDS dementia complex in 1989–1990 in Italy: possible role of the early treatment with zidovudine. Medicina (Firenze) 10:415–416, 1990

Chiesi A, Vella S, Dally LG, et al: Epidemiology of AIDS dementia complex in Europe. AIDS in Europe Study Group. J Acquir Immune Defic Syndr Hum Retrovirol 11:39–44, 1996

Fischl MA, Daikos GL, Uttamchandani RB, et al: The efficacy of azidothymidine (AZT) in the treatment of patients with AIDS and AIDS-related complex. N Engl J Med 317:185–191, 1987

Lyketsos CG, Hanson A, Fishman M, et al: Screening for psychiatric morbidity in a medical outpatient clinic for HIV infection: the need for a psychiatric presence. Int J Psychiatry Med 24:103–113, 1994

Lyketsos CG, Hoover DR, Guccione M, et al: Changes in depressive symptoms as AIDS develops. Am J Psychiatry 153:1430–1437, 1996

Portegies P, De Gans J, Lange JM, et al: Declining incidence of AIDS dementia complex after introduction of zidovudine treatment. BMJ 299:819–821, 1989 (published erratum appears in BMJ 299:1141, 1989)

Sidtis JJ, Gatsonis C, Price RW, et al (for the AIDS Clinical Trials Group): Zidovudine treatment of the AIDS dementia complex: results of a placebo-controlled trial. Ann Neurol 33:343–349, 1993

Tozzi V, Narciso P, Galgani S, et al: Effects of zidovudine in 30 patients with mild to end-stage AIDS dementia complex. AIDS 7:683–692, 1993

Vion-Dury J, Nicoli F, Salvan AM, et al: Reversal of brain metabolic alterations with zidovudine detected by proton localized magnetic resonance spectroscopy (letter). Lancet 345:60–61, 1995

# CHAPTER 29

# Dermatology

*Select the single best response for each question.*

29.1  Atopic dermatitis is an often-chronic clinical problem with meaningful psychiatric comorbidity. Which of the following statements is *not* true?

  A.  Emotional distress aggravates the symptom of pruritis in Alzheimer's disease patients with atopic dermatitis.
  B.  Psychiatric comorbidity in atopic dermatitis is sufficiently common to warrant recommendation for routine psychiatric consultation.
  C.  Various behavioral therapy models have been shown to reduce anxiety and depression in patients with atopic dermatitis.
  D.  Topical doxepin cream has been shown to decrease itching in atopic dermatitis.
  E.  Trimipramine has been shown to reduce nighttime scratching by increasing the time spent in stage I sleep.

**The correct response is option E.**

Trimipramine, an antidepressant with histamine receptor antagonism, decreases the fragmentation of sleep and reduces the time spent in stage I sleep, which in turn diminishes the amount of scratching that occurs during the night (Savin et al. 1979). **(pp. 630–631)**

29.2  Psoriasis is a chronic and relapsing dermatological disease of major importance to the psychiatrist, both because the disease is associated with significant psychiatric comorbidity and because it can occur as a side effect of psychiatric treatment. Which of the following statements is *true*?

  A.  Lithium-induced psoriasis typically persists after lithium is discontinued.
  B.  Bipolar patients who suffer from psoriasis due to lithium treatment should also avoid valproate, because of its similar risk for psoriasis.
  C.  Psoriasis patients have been shown to be at high risk for comorbid personality disorders, including schizoid and avoidant personality disorders.
  D.  Disability from psoriasis is more strongly correlated with disease severity and location than with psychosocial variables.
  E.  Introduction of corticosteroids is correlated with triggering of psoriasis, but withdrawal of corticosteroids is not.

**The correct response is option C.**

Patients with psoriasis have been shown to have high levels of anxiety and depression and significant comorbidity with several personality disorders, including schizoid, avoidant, passive-aggressive, and compulsive personality disorders.

  Lithium-induced psoriasis resolves after discontinuation of lithium. Valproate and carbamazepine are less likely than lithium to exacerbate psoriasis in bipolar disorder. Psychological factors are stronger determinants of disability in patients with psoriasis than are disease severity, location, and duration. Common triggers of psoriasis include cold weather, physical trauma, acute bacterial and viral infections, corticosteroid withdrawal, beta-adrenergic blockers, and lithium. **(p. 631)**

29.3   Delusional parasitosis is an unusual syndrome in which the patient believes that he or she is infested with living organisms. Which of the following is *not* true?

A. Patients typically have experienced a specific precipitating event.
B. Patients typically have had actual exposure to parasites.
C. Patients usually readily accept psychiatric referral.
D. Affected patients often respond to treatment with pimozide.
E. QT prolongation from pimozide limits its use in patients with dysrhythmias.

**The correct response is option C.**

Many patients are reluctant to accept psychiatric evaluation for fear of being told that the infestation is not real. A specific precipitant, "actual" exposure to contagious organisms or infestation, and resistance to psychiatric evaluation are common. Pimozide, a neuroleptic, has demonstrated positive effects in patients with delusional parasitosis. **(p. 635)**

29.4   Psychogenic excoriation may lead to substantial dermatological problems. Depressive and anxiety disorders are common in patients with this condition. Case reports and small open trials have shown some efficacy for psychotropic medications in psychogenic excoriation. Which two tricyclic antidepressants (TCAs) have been shown to be effective?

A. Nortriptyline and doxepin.
B. Doxepin and clomipramine.
C. Nortriptyline and desipramine.
D. Imipramine and doxepin.
E. Imipramine and desipramine.

**The correct response is option B.**

The TCAs doxepin (Harris et al. 1987) and clomipramine (Gupta et al. 1986) have been shown to be effective for psychogenic excoriation, as have several selective serotonin reuptake inhibitors and antipsychotics. **(p. 636)**

29.5   Which of the following is *not* true of trichotillomania or its psychiatric comorbidity?

A. The mean age at onset of trichotillomania is after age 15 years.
B. Anxiety, mood, and substance use disorders are commonly comorbid with trichotillomania.
C. The comorbid personality disorders most frequently seen with trichotillomania are the Cluster B and Cluster C personality disorders.
D. First-degree relatives of affected patients have high rates of obsessive-compulsive disorder.
E. Clomipramine has been shown to be superior to desipramine for treatment, supporting an "obsessive-compulsive spectrum" construct for trichotillomania.

**The correct response is option A.**

The mean age at onset of trichotillomania is 13 years.

   Comorbid psychiatric disorders in patients with trichotillomania include anxiety, mood, substance abuse, and eating disorders. No particular personality disorder is characteristic of patients with trichotillomania (Christenson et al. 1992), although a family history of obsessive-compulsive disorder and trichotillomania is common (Swedo and Leonard 1992). In one study, trichotillomania showed a better response to clomipramine than to desipramine (Swedo et al. 1989). **(p. 637)**

29.6     Lithium is notoriously associated with a range of dermatological side effects, which may limit its use. Lithium's dermatological side effects commonly include all of the following *except*

    A.   Skin pigmentation.
    B.   Urticaria.
    C.   Alopecia.
    D.   Psoriasis.
    E.   Exacerbation of acne.

**The correct response is option A.**

Skin pigmentation is a side effect not of lithium but of antipsychotics. Lithium's dermatological side effects include urticaria, rash, alopecia, folliculitis, exacerbation of acne, and psoriasis. **(p. 640, Table 29–3)**

# References

Christenson GA, Chernoff-Clementz E, Clementz BA: Personality and clinical characteristics in patients with trichotillomania. J Clin Psychiatry 53:407–413, 1992

Harris BA, Sherertz EF, Flowers FP: Improvement of chronic neurotic excoriations with oral doxepin therapy. Int J Dermatol 26:541–543, 1987

Gupta MA, Gupta AK, Haberman HF: Neurotic excoriations: a review and some new perspectives. Compr Psychiatry 27:381–386, 1986

Savin JA, Paterson WD, Adam K, et al: Effects of trimeprazine and trimipramine on nocturnal scratching in patients with atopic eczema. Arch Dermatol 115:313–315, 1979

Swedo SE, Leonard HL: Trichotillomania: an obsessive compulsive spectrum disorder? Psychiatr Clin North Am 15:777–790, 1992

Swedo SE, Leonard HL, Rapoport JL, et al: A double-blind comparison of clomipramine and desipramine in the treatment of trichotillomania (hair pulling). N Engl J Med 321:497–501, 1989

# CHAPTER 30

# Surgery

*Select the single best response for each question.*

30.1 Which of the following are the elements of informed consent that a surgeon should include in his or her discussion with a patient about a proposed surgery?

A. Diagnosis.
B. Why the surgery is the treatment of choice.
C. Expected risks and benefits.
D. Alternatives and their consequences.
E. All of the above.

**The correct response is option E.**

The communication of factual information understandable to the patient is the responsibility of the surgeon. It should include diagnosis, reasons that the operation is thought to be the treatment of choice, and expected risks and benefits and their probabilities. Alternatives and their consequences, as well as financial costs, also should be discussed. Competent patients have a right to decide whether to accept or reject a proposed surgery. Although the psychiatric consultant cannot legally declare a patient incompetent, he or she can evaluate the medicolegal elements of the patient's decision-making capacity. **(p. 649)**

30.2 What percentage of children experience significant preoperative anxiety?

A. Less than 10%.
B. 10%–20%.
C. 40%–60%.
D. 80%–90%.
E. None of the above.

**The correct response is option C.**

It is estimated that as many as 3 million children undergo anesthesia and surgery annually in the United States. Many children (40%–60%) experience significant anxiety before surgery. It has been postulated that postoperative outcome may be influenced by preoperative anxiety. **(p. 651)**

30.3 Risk factors for developing postoperative delirium include all of the following *except*

A. Older age.
B. Alcohol use.
C. Cognitive impairment.
D. Male gender.
E. Type of surgery.

**The correct response is option D.**

Multiple preoperative risk factors for postoperative delirium have been identified and include older age, alcohol use, cognitive impairment (especially the dementias), chronic comorbid illnesses and medications used to treat these illnesses, severity of the acute illness, and type of surgery. Postoperative changes in the sleep–wake cycle, inadequately treated pain, and use of medications such as benzodiazepines increase the likelihood of delirium. **(p. 653)**

30.4   Which psychiatric disorder has been found in burn patients during all phases (resuscitative, acute, and convalescent) of injury?

   A.  Delirium.
   B.  Posttraumatic stress disorder.
   C.  Alcohol abuse.
   D.  Mood disorder.
   E.  Cognitive disorder.

**The correct response is option B.**

Posttraumatic stress disorder is found during all phases of injury in burn patients. Delirium and cognitive disorder are present in the resuscitative phase; mood disorder, in both the acute and the convalescent phases; and alcohol abuse, in the convalescent phase. **(p. 658, Table 30–1)**

30.5   Bariatric surgery is usually performed for patients with extreme or morbid obesity. According to the National Heart, Lung, and Blood Institute guidelines, *extreme obesity* is a body mass index (BMI) of

   A.  $>15$ kg/m$^2$.
   B.  $>20$ kg/m$^2$.
   C.  $>25$ kg/m$^2$.
   D.  $>30$ kg/m$^2$.
   E.  $>40$ kg/m$^2$.

**The correct response is option E.**

The National Heart, Lung, and Blood Institute (1998) clinical guidelines define extreme obesity as a BMI greater than 40 kg/m$^2$. BMI is a calculated number attained by dividing weight in kilograms by height in meters squared. Extreme obesity is also called morbid obesity because it is associated with high premature morbidity and mortality, most commonly as a result of complications of type 2 diabetes mellitus, hypertension, hyperlipidemia, or sleep apnea. **(p. 664)**

# Reference

National Heart, Lung, and Blood Institute: Clinical Guidelines on the Identification, Evaluation, and Treatment of Overweight and Obesity in Adults. Bethesda, MD, National Institutes of Health, National Heart, Lung, and Blood Institute, June 1998

# CHAPTER 31

# Organ Transplantation

*Select the single best response for each question.*

31.1 Which of the following organ transplantations has the highest percentage of patient survival at 10 years posttransplant?

A. Lung.
B. Kidney.
C. Pancreas.
D. Heart.
E. Liver.

**The correct response is option C.**

Pancreas transplant recipients have the highest percentage of survival at 10 years posttransplant, a survival rate of approximately 70%. **(p. 677, Figure 31–3)**

31.2 Psychosocial rating instruments may be of value in assessing patients' psychological preparation for and adaptation to transplant surgery. All of the following are true *except*

A. The Psychosocial Assessment of Candidates for Transplantation (PACT) provides both an overall score and a series of subscale scores.
B. The PACT can be quickly completed but requires scoring by a skilled and experienced clinician.
C. The Transplant Evaluation Rating Scale (TERS) rates 10 discrete areas of psychological functioning.
D. Because the TERS has more scored items than the PACT, it is more appealing as a research tool.
E. Between the two instruments, the TERS is considered to be more flexible than the PACT in terms of clinical use.

**The correct response is option E.**

The PACT is considered to be more flexible than the TERS, both in the range of rating individual items and in the manner in which the summary score is determined. **(p. 679)**

31.3 Factors that increase the risk of posttransplantation psychiatric illness include all of the following *except*

A. Pretransplant history of psychiatric illness.
B. Longer hospitalization.
C. Male gender.
D. Greater physical impairment.
E. Fewer social supports.

**The correct response is option C.**

*Female gender*, not male gender, is one of the factors that increases the risk of posttransplantation psychiatric illness. **(pp. 680–681)**

31.4 Psychiatric disorders may have an impact on the posttransplant health outcomes of patients. Which of the following statements is *true*?

    A. Liver transplant candidates with Beck Depression Inventory (BDI) scores greater than 10 were more likely than nondepressed candidates to die while awaiting transplantation.

    B. In liver disease patients with high BDI scores, the higher scores are attributable to a greater number of somatic symptoms.

    C. In liver transplant candidates who receive transplantation, high pretransplant BDI scores predict poorer posttransplant survival.

    D. In heart transplant patients, posttraumatic stress disorder (PTSD) related to the transplant surgery itself was not associated with a higher mortality rate.

    E. Lung transplant patients without a presurgical psychiatric history were more likely to survive 1 year postsurgery compared with those with a psychiatric history.

**The correct response is option A.**

Liver transplant candidates with BDI scores greater than 10 (64% of patients) were significantly more likely than nondepressed candidates to die while awaiting transplantation (Singh et al. 1997). The higher BDI scores were due more to psychological distress than to somatic symptoms. However, for candidates who reached transplantation, pretransplant depression was not associated with poorer posttransplant survival (Singh et al. 1997).

    In a study of 191 heart transplant recipients, PTSD (with the traumatic event being transplant-related) was associated with higher mortality (Dew and Kormos 1999). A study of lung transplant recipients found that those with a pretransplant psychiatric history were more likely than those without such a history to be alive 1 year after transplantation (Woodman et al. 1999). **(pp. 680–681)**

31.5 Because of the complexity of posttransplant immunosuppressive and other ongoing medical therapy, treatment compliance is crucial to the ongoing well-being of these patients. Which of the following statements is *not* true?

    A. Medical noncompliance in posttransplant patients is estimated at 20%–50%.

    B. Noncompliance is a major risk factor for graft rejection and may account for 25% of deaths after the initial recovery period.

    C. In the Dew study of compliance in heart transplant recipients (Dew et al. 1996), nonadherence to immunosuppressive medication regimens was the most frequent area of noncompliance.

    D. Persisting psychiatric illness after transplantation is associated with medical noncompliance.

    E. A "dose–response" relationship between number of risk factors present and rates of noncompliance predicts higher rates of noncompliance with more risk factors.

**The correct response is option C.**

Dew and colleagues (1996) examined compliance in eight domains of posttransplant care. The degree of noncompliance varied, but noncompliance was most persistent in the domains of exercise (37%), blood pressure monitoring (34%), immunosuppressive medication (20%), smoking (19%), diet (18%), blood work completion (15%), clinic attendance (9%), and heavy drinking (6%). **(p. 683)**

31.6    As is true in other areas of medical practice in which a high degree of personal investment in care is required for a successful sense of physician–patient collaboration, patients with personality disorders present special challenges for the multidisciplinary transplant team. Which of the following personality disorders is associated with the highest rate of posttransplant noncompliance?

A. Obsessive-compulsive.
B. Borderline.
C. Antisocial.
D. Narcissistic.
E. Avoidant.

**The correct response is option B.**

Borderline personality disorder is considered to represent the highest risk for posttransplant noncompliance. **(pp. 686–687)**


31.7    Hepatic encephalopathy is a neuropsychiatric illness associated with end-stage liver disease that frequently comes to the attention of the psychosomatic medicine specialist. Which of the following is *not* true of hepatic encephalopathy?

A. Alteration of consciousness and cognitive impairment are common in hepatic encephalopathy.
B. Additional psychological tests (e.g., the Trail Making Test) may facilitate diagnosis in more subtle cases.
C. A major focus of treatment is to reduce the production and absorption of ammonia from the gastrointestinal tract.
D. Serum ammonia levels correlate well with degree of neuropsychiatric symptoms.
E. Anticholinergic medications should be stopped or avoided in hepatic encephalopathy.

**The correct response is option D.**

Treatment should be targeted toward reducing serum ammonia levels, even though serum ammonia levels are *not* well correlated with symptoms of hepatic encephalopathy (Riordan and Williams 1997). Alteration of consciousness and cognitive impairment are characteristic symptoms of the illness. Anticholinergic drugs, tranquilizers, and sedatives should be avoided in hepatic encephalopathy. **(p. 688)**

# References

Dew M, Kormos R: Early posttransplant medical compliance and mental health predict physical morbidity and mortality one to three years after heart transplantation. J Heart Lung Transplant 18:549–562, 1999

Dew MA, Roth LH, Thompson ME, et al: Medical compliance and its predictors in the first year after heart transplantation. J Heart Lung Transplant 15:631–645, 1996

Riordan SM, Williams R: Treatment of hepatic encephalopathy. N Engl J Med 337:473–479, 1997

Singh N, Gayowski T, Wagener MM, et al: Depression in patients with cirrhosis: impact on outcome. Dig Dis Sci 42:1421–1427, 1997

Woodman CL, Geist LJ, Vance S, et al: Psychiatric disorders and survival after lung transplantation. Psychosomatics 40:293–297, 1999

# CHAPTER 3 2

# Neurology and Neurosurgery

*Select the single best response for each question.*

32.1   The classic clinical presentation of middle cerebral artery infarction in the dominant hemisphere includes all of the following *except*

    A.  Contralateral hemiparesis.
    B.  Neglect.
    C.  Aphasia.
    D.  Sensory loss of a cortical type.
    E.  None of the above.

**The correct response is option B.**

Lesions in the nondominant hemisphere may be accompanied by neglect or perceptual disturbance.

    The classic presentation of middle cerebral artery infarction is contralateral hemiparesis and sensory loss of a cortical type. These are often accompanied by hemianopsia if the optic radiation is affected. If the lesion is in the dominant hemisphere, then aphasia may be expected. **(p. 702)**

32.2   Which of the following is a category or type of vascular dementia?

    A.  Subcortical ischemic dementia.
    B.  Multi-infarct dementia.
    C.  Dementia due to focal "strategic" infarction.
    D.  A and B.
    E.  A, B, and C.

**The correct response is option E.**

*Vascular dementia* is an imprecise term referring to a heterogeneous group of dementing disorders caused by impairment of the brain's blood supply. These disorders fall into three principal categories: subcortical ischemic dementia, multi-infarct dementia, and dementia due to focal "strategic" infarction. Several sets of diagnostic criteria are available, with high specificity but low sensitivity for pathologically defined vascular dementia (Chui et al. 1992; Hachinski et al. 1974; Roman et al. 1993). **(p. 702)**

32.3   Which of the following are core features of Parkinson's disease?

    A.  Tremor.
    B.  Rigidity.
    C.  Bradykinesia.
    D.  None of the above.
    E.  A, B, and C.

The correct response is option E.

The core feature of Parkinson's disease is the triad of tremor, rigidity, and bradykinesia (Sethi 2002). Bradykinesia—usually of insidious onset and easily misdiagnosed as depression or boredom—is the most common first sign and ultimately is the most disabling symptom. Resting tremor is the most characteristic feature of Parkinson's disease, affecting more than 70% of patients. In the early stages of the disease, the tremor is described as "pill-rolling." The rigidity manifests as fixed abnormalities of posture and resistance to passive movement throughout the range of motion. (p. 706)

32.4    Pathologically, multiple sclerosis is characterized by all of the following *except*

   A. Loss of oligodendrocytes.
   B. Astroglial scarring.
   C. Microhemorrhages.
   D. Multifocal areas of demyelination.
   E. Relative preservation of axons.

The correct response is option C.

Microhemorrhages are *not* characteristic of multiple sclerosis. Pathologically, multiple sclerosis is characterized by multifocal areas of demyelination with relative preservation of axons, loss of oligodendrocytes, and astroglial scarring. Although axons are relatively spared, axonal loss and cortical atrophy occur. (p. 707)

32.5    Which of the following statements concerning Huntington's disease is *true*?

   A. Has a prevalence rate of 5–7 per 100,000 population.
   B. Affects men more than women.
   C. The most common age at onset is in young or middle adulthood.
   D. A and C.
   E. A, B, and C.

The correct response is option D.

Huntington's disease occurs at a prevalence of 5–7 per 100,000 population in the United States, with wide regional variations. Onset can be at any age but most commonly is in young or middle adulthood. The sexes are affected equally. The disorder exhibits the phenomenon of *anticipation*, in which the age at onset tends to decrease over the generations, especially with paternal transmission. (p. 710)

32.6    The brain region most commonly activated during partial seizures is the

   A. Temporal lobe.
   B. Parietal lobe.
   C. Occipital lobe.
   D. Frontal lobe.
   E. None of the above.

The correct response is option A.

Seizures affecting the temporal lobe can be the most difficult to diagnose, but this lobe is also the most common site of onset, accounting for 80% of partial seizures. Symptoms may include auditory hallucinations, ranging from simple sounds to complex language.

Seizures originating in the parietal lobe can cause tingling or numbness in a bodily region or more complex sensory experiences such as a sense of absence on one side of the body, or asomatognosia. Seizures of the occipital lobe are associated with visual symptoms, which are usually elementary (e.g., simple flashing lights). Complex partial seizures of frontal lobe origin tend to begin and end abruptly, with minimal postictal confusion. **(pp. 714–715)**

# References

Chui HC, Victoroff JI, Margolin D: Criteria for the diagnosis of ischemic vascular dementia proposed by the State of California Alzheimer Disease Diagnostic and Treatment Centers (ADDTC). Neurology 42:473–480, 1992

Hachinski VC, Lassen NA, Marshall J: Multi-infarct dementia: a cause of mental deterioration in the elderly. Lancet 2 (7874):207–210, 1974

Roman GC, Tatimichi TK, Erkinjuntti T: Vascular dementia: diagnostic criteria for research studies. Report of the NINDS-AIREN International Workshop. Neurology 43:250–260, 1993

Sethi KD: Clinical aspects of Parkinson disease. Curr Opin Neurol 15:457–460, 2002

# C H A P T E R    3 3

# Obstetrics and Gynecology

*Select the single best response for each question.*

33.1    Infertility is a common clinical problem in obstetric/gynecological practice that is often fraught with psychosocial distress. Attention to and management of comorbid psychiatric illness may be an important part of infertility treatment. All of the following statements are true *except*

A.  The prevalence of infertility has increased steadily since 1965.
B.  Generalized anxiety disorder (GAD) is associated with lower rates of fecundity.
C.  A higher trait anxiety level is associated with a lower pregnancy rate.
D.  Comorbid depression is associated with lower pregnancy rates in women undergoing in vitro fertilization.
E.  Infertility is associated with rates of depression similar to those in chronic illnesses (e.g., heart disease, cancer).

**The correct response is option A.**

The rate of infertility has remained relatively stable since 1965, although the popular impression is that it has risen.

GAD is associated with lower rates of fertility (King 2003); trait anxiety is associated with lower pregnancy rates (Demyttenaere et al. 1988). Depression is associated with lower pregnancy rates after in vitro fertilization (Demyttenaere et al. 1998). **(p. 734)**


33.2    The pharmacological interactions between psychotropic medications and contraceptives may result in unwelcome clinical events. All of the following statements are true *except*

A.  Implanted levonorgestrel metabolism can be enhanced by phenobarbital, decreasing contraceptive effectiveness.
B.  Oral contraceptives inhibit the metabolism of tricyclic antidepressants, thus increasing serum levels.
C.  Oral contraceptives enhance the metabolism of benzodiazepines, decreasing their effectiveness.
D.  Modafinil increases the metabolism of oral contraceptives.
E.  Carbamazepine and oxcarbazepine both enhance the metabolism of oral contraceptives.

**The correct response is option C.**

Oral contraceptives inhibit the hepatic oxidation of benzodiazepines and tricyclic antidepressants, thus enhancing their effectiveness. By contrast, modafinil, carbamazepine, and oxcarbazepine enhance the metabolism of oral contraceptives, thereby decreasing their effectiveness. **(p. 736)**

33.3 Hysterectomy is a common gynecological procedure that frequently involves significant psychiatric factors. Which of the following statements is *true*?

    A. Because it is associated with less surgical mortality, vaginal hysterectomy is now more common than abdominal hysterectomy.

    B. Among women who undergo hysterectomy, African American women have the procedure at an older age than do other American women, on the average.

    C. Women who undergo hysterectomy for chronic pelvic pain have better psychological outcomes than do women who undergo hysterectomy for bleeding.

    D. Women undergoing surgical hysterectomy with oophorectomy are at risk for depression, especially if they have a history of depression associated with reproductive events.

    E. Most studies show a decrease in sexuality in women following hysterectomy.

**The correct response is option D.**

Women undergoing hysterectomy with oophorectomy are subject to sudden surgical menopause and are at risk for depression, especially if they have a history of depression associated with reproductive events.

    Although vaginal hysterectomies are associated with less surgical mortality and shorter lengths of stay, abdominal hysterectomies are still more commonly performed. African American women, on the average, undergo hysterectomy at a younger age. Women who have hysterectomy for chronic pelvic pain have worse psychological outcomes than do women who have the procedure because of bleeding. Most studies have found no change in sexuality in women following hysterectomy. **(pp. 737–738)**

33.4 Chronic pelvic pain is an obstetric/gynecological condition associated with significant psychiatric comorbidity. Which of the following statements is *not* true?

    A. Other somatic symptoms are common in chronic pelvic pain.

    B. Patients with chronic pelvic pain frequently have a history of physical and/or sexual abuse.

    C. The explanatory model of "psychogenic pain," wherein emotional pain is "displaced" onto the body, remains the most useful construct in understanding chronic pelvic pain.

    D. Mood and anxiety disorders are common in patients with chronic pelvic pain.

    E. Psychiatric diagnoses have been reported in 60% of these patients.

**The correct response is option C.**

The concept of "psychogenic pain" has been largely superseded, and we have moved increasingly toward multicausal views of chronic pelvic pain.

    Most studies have reported more depression, somatic symptoms, substance abuse, sexual dysfunction, and physical and sexual abuse in patients with chronic pelvic pain than in comparison groups. Mood and anxiety disorders, marital adjustment problems, spousal responses, abuse history, and somatization have been reported in 60% of these patients. **(p. 740)**

33.5 Psychiatric disorders that occur during pregnancy can be of great concern because of the challenges of managing a pregnant psychiatric patient. Which of the following statements is *true*?

    A. Panic disorder patients who become pregnant should continue on medication throughout pregnancy.

    B. Obsessive-compulsive disorder is likely to worsen postpartum but not prepartum.

    C. Electroconvulsive therapy (ECT) for acute psychosis during pregnancy can be effective and is generally safe for the fetus.

D. Despite the later-appearing cognitive impairments, the perinatal mortality for fetal alcohol syndrome is less than 5%.

E. In "crack babies," the cognitive impairments are usually due to the toxic exposure to cocaine in utero rather than to social factors.

**The correct response is option C.**

ECT for acute affective psychotic episodes can be effective and is relatively safe for the fetus.

Patients with panic disorder should be tapered off medication gradually and treated with cognitive-behavioral therapy. Obsessive-compulsive disorder is likely to worsen both pre- and postpartum. The perinatal mortality for fetal alcohol syndrome is 17%. Most of the negative cognitive and behavioral findings in "crack babies" appear to result from the environment in which they grow up rather than from intrauterine exposure to cocaine. **(pp. 742–743)**

33.6 Postpartum depression and psychosis are among the most serious and potentially dangerous conditions in psychiatry because of their threat to infant safety. Which of the following statements is *true*?

A. Miscarriage increases the risk of depression in subsequent pregnancies, but stillbirth does not.

B. Postpartum depression incidence in North America is 30%–40% of pregnancies.

C. Thyroxine administration has been shown to decrease the risk of postpartum depression.

D. Antecedent anxiety disorder is a more important risk factor for postpartum depression than is antecedent depression.

E. Relatives of a patient with postpartum depression should typically offer to assume total care of the newborn.

**The correct response is option D.**

Antecedent anxiety disorder has been found to be a more important risk factor for postpartum depression than is antecedent depression (Matthey et al. 2003).

Stillbirths, as well as miscarriages, increase the risk of posttraumatic stress, anxiety, and depression in a subsequent pregnancy. Postpartum depression occurs in up to 10%–20% of mothers in North America. Thyroxine administration does not appear to reduce the risk of postpartum depression. Relatives should not offer to assume total care of the newborn, because doing so would only exacerbate the mother's sense of failure and deprivation; rather, they should offer to help with household tasks, allow her to care for the infant, and reinforce her sense of maternal adequacy. **(pp. 744–745)**

# References

Demyttenaere K, Nijs P, Steeno O, et al: Anxiety and conception rates in donor insemination. J Psychosom Obstet Gynaecol 8:175–181, 1988

Demyttenaere K, Bonte L, Gheldof M, et al: Coping style and depression level influence outcome in vitro fertilization. Fertil Steril 69:1026–1033, 1998

King R: Subfecundity and anxiety in a nationally representative sample. Soc Sci Med 56:739–751, 2003

Matthey S, Barnett B, Howie P, et al: Diagnosing postpartum depression in mothers and fathers: whatever happened to anxiety? J Affect Disord 74:139–147, 2003

# CHAPTER 34

# Pediatrics

*Select the single best response for each question.*

34.1    Which of the following is *not* one of Piaget's stages of cognitive development?

   A.  Concrete operations.
   B.  Informal operations.
   C.  Sensorimotor operations.
   D.  Preoperational thought.
   E.  Formal operations.

**The correct response is option B.**

Informal operations is not a Piagetian stage.

   Children appear to follow a developmental path of understanding their bodies that roughly corresponds to Piaget's stages of cognitive development. *Sensorimotor* children (birth to approximately 2 years) are largely preverbal and do not have the capacity to create narratives to explain their experiences. Their perception of their bodies and of illness is therefore primarily built on sensory experiences and does not involve any formal reasoning. *Preoperational* children (approximately 2–7 years) also understand through perception, but they are able to use words and some very basic concepts of cause and effect. They tend to be most aware of parts of the body that they can directly sense, such as bones and heart (which they can feel) and blood (which they have seen come out of their bodies). They also have no real sense of organs, but instead conceptualize blood and food as going into or coming out of their bodies as though the body were itself the container. This leads to many humorous but confusing assumptions and misunderstandings. *Concrete operational* children (approximately 7–11 years) are able to apply logic to their perceptions. However, the logic is quite literal or concrete and allows for only one cause for an effect. Children tend to be eager to learn factual information about the body and illness at this age, but they will have difficulty with any concepts that require abstract reasoning. *Formal operational* children (11+ years) are able to use a level of abstract reasoning that allows discussion of systems rather than simple organs and can incorporate multiple causations of illness. It should not be assumed, however, that all adolescents approach the understanding of illness and their bodies at this level of cognition. **(p. 761)**

34.2    Which of the following statements concerning failure to thrive (FTT) children is *incorrect*?

   A.  Feeding problems and growth deficiencies can occur.
   B.  Mothers of FTT children are reported to have experienced high rates of physical abuse.
   C.  If a FTT child gains weight in the hospital, a psychosocial cause of the FTT should be presumed.
   D.  Former FTT children have more behavioral problems than do children without a history of FTT.
   E.  None of the above.

**The correct response is option C.**

Some FTT children who have an inadequate caregiver will still lose weight in the hospital, simply because they are separated from the caregiver.

In one study of FTT children (who had no identifiable biological contributors), 80% of the mothers reported a history of physical abuse (Weston et al. 1993). Former FTT children have been found to be smaller, less cognitively able, and more behaviorally disturbed than children without a history of FTT, especially if their mothers are poorly educated (Drewett et al. 1999; Dykman et al. 2001). (p. 767)

34.3   Which of the following statements about cystic fibrosis is *correct?*

A.  It occurs in approximately one of every 100,000 live Caucasian births.
B.  It affects approximately 250,000 children and adults in the United States.
C.  Less than 10% of patients with cystic fibrosis are adults.
D.  Eighty percent of patients with cystic fibrosis are diagnosed by age 3 years.
E.  None of the above.

**The correct response is option D.**

More than 80% of cystic fibrosis patients are diagnosed by age 3 years; however, almost 10% are diagnosed at age 18 years or older.

A defective gene causes the body to produce a thick, sticky mucus that clogs the lungs and leads to life-threatening lung infections. These secretions also obstruct the pancreas, preventing digestive enzymes from reaching the intestines. Cystic fibrosis affects approximately 30,000 children and adults in the United States and is the most common hereditary disease in white children. Cystic fibrosis has a prevalence of approximately 1 per 3,200 live Caucasian births, with about 1,000 new cases diagnosed each year. (p. 770)

34.4   Vocal cord dysfunction

A.  Commonly occurs comorbidly with asthma.
B.  Is often associated with anxiety.
C.  Can mimic asthma.
D.  Is associated with chronic stress.
E.  All of the above.

**The correct response is option E.**

Vocal cord dysfunction can mimic asthma and commonly occurs comorbidly with asthma. It is a condition of involuntary paradoxical adduction of the vocal cords during the inspiratory phase of the respiratory cycle. It is often associated with anxiety or chronic stress; however, sexual abuse in this population is not as prevalent as was previously believed (Brugman et al. 1994; Gavin et al. 1998). Patients with vocal cord dysfunction frequently present with stridulous breathing, experience tightness in their throats, and feel short of breath. It can be quite worrisome that the symptoms are unrelieved by asthma medications. (p. 771)

34.5   Which of the following statements concerning childhood obesity is *incorrect?*

A.  Children are considered obese if they have a body mass index (BMI) greater than or equal to the 95th percentile for age and gender.
B.  Recent data from the third Natural Health and Nutrition Examination Survey, conducted from 1988 to 1994, indicated that approximately 11% of U.S. children are obese.
C.  Increases in childhood obesity have not been documented in Asia.

D. Children with a BMI at or above the 95th percentile for age and gender have significantly reduced health-related quality of life.
E. Obese adolescents are less likely to complete college than are nonoverweight adolescents of similar educational backgrounds.

**The correct response is option C.**

Increases in childhood obesity equivalent to those registered in the United States have been documented in Asia and Europe.

There has been a disturbing increase during the past 20 years in the prevalence of obesity in children and adolescents in the United States. Data from the third National Health and Nutrition Examination Survey, conducted from 1988 to 1994, indicated that approximately 11% of children were obese and another 14% were overweight (Troiano et al. 1995). The impact of obesity is both immediate and long-lasting. Children and adolescents with a BMI at or above the 95th percentile for age and sex are considered obese; they have been found to have significantly reduced health-related quality of life compared with healthy children and adolescents. In a study of 106 children, ages 5–18 years, the obese subjects were more than five times more likely to have significant impairment of physical functioning and almost six times as likely to have impaired psychosocial health. A survey of approximately 10,000 women, ages 16–24 years, found that obese adolescents were less likely to complete college than were nonoverweight adolescents of similar educational backgrounds. **(p. 772)**

# References

Brugman SM, Howell JH, Mahler JL, et al: The spectrum of pediatric vocal cord dysfunction. Am Rev Respir Dis 149:A353, 1994

Drewett RF, Corbett SS, Wright CM: Cognitive and educational attainments at school age of children who failed to thrive in infancy: a population-based study. J Child Psychol Psychiatry 40:551–561, 1999

Dykman RA, Casey PH, Ackerman PT, et al: Behavioral and cognitive status in school-aged children with a history of failure to thrive during early childhood. Clin Pediatr (Phila) 40:63–70, 2001

Gavin LA, Wamboldt M, Brugman S, et al: Psychological and family characteristics of adolescents with vocal cord dysfunction. J Asthma 35:409–417, 1998

Troiano RP, Flegal KM, Kuczmarski RJ, et al: Overweight prevalence and trends for children and adolescents: the National Health and Nutrition Examination Surveys, 1963 to 1991. Arch Pediatr Adolesc Med 149:1085–1091, 1995

Weston JA, Colloton M, Halsey S, et al: A legacy of violence in nonorganic failure to thrive. Child Abuse Negl 17:709–714, 1993

# CHAPTER 35

# Physical Medicine and Rehabilitation

*Select the single best response for each question.*

35.1   Which of the following is considered a less significant risk factor for psychiatric illness following traumatic brain injury (TBI)?

A.  Poor neuropsychological functioning.
B.  Preinjury psychiatric history.
C.  Preinjury social impairment.
D.  Increased age.
E.  Alcohol abuse.

**The correct response is option A.**

Poor neuropsychological functioning is a less significant risk factor for psychiatric illness following TBI, whereas preinjury psychiatric history, preinjury social impairment, increased age, alcohol abuse, and arteriosclerosis are highly significant risk factors. **(pp. 790–791, Table 35–2)**

35.2   Regarding post-TBI psychosis, which of the following statements is *true*?

A.  In TBI-associated psychosis, hallucinations are more commonly reported than are delusions.
B.  Right-hemisphere lesions are more common than left-sided lesions in TBI-associated psychosis.
C.  Seizure disorder rates in patients with post-TBI psychosis are higher than estimates for rates of post-TBI seizure disorders in general.
D.  The onset of psychotic symptoms is typically within 3 months of injury, with delayed onset after 1 year rarely reported.
E.  Negative symptoms are more common in post-TBI psychosis than are positive symptoms.

**The correct response is option C.**

Rates of seizure disorders in patients with psychosis after TBI have been found to be much higher than estimates for rates of seizure disorders after TBI in general (Fujii and Ahmed 2002).

Delusions, most commonly persecutory, are much more common than hallucinations. Risk factors for psychosis include left-hemisphere and temporal lobe lesions, closed head injury, and increasing severity of TBI. The onset of psychotic symptoms is typically gradual and delayed, often occurring more than 1 year after injury. Auditory hallucinations and paranoid delusions are more common than negative symptoms. **(pp. 794–795)**

35.3 All of the following are considered risk factors for postconcussive syndrome *except*

    A. Older age.
    B. Previous TBI.
    C. Psychosocial stress.
    D. Male gender.
    E. Ongoing litigation.

**The correct response is option D.**

Male gender is not a risk factor for postconcussive syndrome. The more common risk factors are female gender, older age, history of previous TBI, psychosocial stress, poor social support, low socioeconomic status, and presence of ongoing litigation. **(p. 799)**

35.4 Numerous psychotropic medications can be used to treat the symptoms of apathy and fatigue in central nervous system injury. Which of the following medications used for this purpose carries a risk of inducing seizures at usual doses?

    A. Modafinil.
    B. Methylphenidate.
    C. Dextroamphetamine.
    D. Bromocriptine.
    E. Amantadine.

**The correct response is option E.**

Amantadine has been associated with an increased risk of seizures, but methylphenidate, dextroamphetamine, and bromocriptine do not seem to lower the seizure threshold at typical doses. **(p. 808)**

35.5 Which anticonvulsant/mood stabilizer has been associated with paradoxical agitation in TBI and should thus be used with some caution and careful monitoring?

    A. Oxcarbazepine.
    B. Topiramate.
    C. Valproate.
    D. Lithium.
    E. Gabapentin.

**The correct response is option E.**

Some TBI patients may experience paradoxical agitation with gabapentin (Childers and Holland 1997). This side effect has not been reported with any other medications. **(p. 810)**

35.6 The use of atypical antipsychotic agents in TBI may be helpful in controlling problematic psychotic and agitation symptoms. However, TBI patients are prone to delirium from anticholinergic drug effects and may also have an increased risk of seizures. For these reasons, which of the following antipsychotics should be used only with extreme caution in this population?

    A. Clozapine.
    B. Olanzapine.
    C. Risperidone.

D. Quetiapine.

E. Ziprasidone.

**The correct response is option A.**

Clozapine carries a risk of seizures and should be used with extreme caution in TBI patients, particularly when compliance is in question. **(pp. 810–811)**

# References

Childers MK, Holland D: Psychomotor agitation following gabapentin use in brain injury. Brain Inj 11:537–540, 1997

Fujii D, Ahmed I: Characteristics of psychotic disorder due to traumatic brain injury: an analysis of case studies in the literature. J Neuropsychiatry Clin Neurosci 14:130–140, 2002

# CHAPTER 36

# Pain

*Select the single best response for each question.*

36.1   The International Association for the Study of Pain (IASP) has defined *pain* as

A. An unpleasant, abnormal sensation that can be spontaneous or evoked.

B. An increased response to a stimulus that is normally painful.

C. An unpleasant sensory and emotional experience associated with actual or potential tissue damage.

D. An abnormal sensation, spontaneous or evoked, that is not unpleasant.

E. None of the above.

**The correct response is option C.**

Pain has been defined by the IASP as "an unpleasant sensory and emotional experience associated with actual or potential tissue damage, or described in terms of such damage" (Merskey et al. 1986, p. S217). **(p. 827)**

36.2   Visual prodromal symptoms, such as scintillating scotomata, are indicative of what type of headache?

A. Classic migraine.

B. Complicated migraine.

C. Constant (transformed) migraine.

D. Common migraine.

E. Hemicrania continua.

**The correct response is option A.**

Common migraine is defined as a unilateral pulsatile headache, which may be associated with other symptoms such as nausea, vomiting, photophobia, and phonophobia (Szirmai 1997). The classic form of migraine adds visual prodromal symptoms such as scintillating scotomata.

Complicated migraine includes focal neurological signs such as cranial nerve palsies and is often described by the name of the primary deficit (e.g., hemiplegic, vestibular, or basilar migraine). Chronic daily headache affects about 5% of the population and encompasses constant (transformed) migraine, chronic tension-type headaches, new-onset daily persistent headache, and hemicrania continua (Lake and Saper 2002). **(p. 830)**

36.3   Which of the following statements concerning low back pain is *true*?

A. Nearly 25% percent of patients with acute low back pain will go on to develop chronic symptoms.

B. The least powerful predictor of chronicity is poor functional status 4 weeks after seeking treatment.

C. Economic and social rewards are not associated with higher levels of disability and depression in patients with chronic back pain.

D. Psychological factors highly correlated with low back pain include distress, depressed mood, and somatization.
E. The presence of an anxiety disorder has been demonstrated to increase the risk of developing chronic musculoskeletal pain 3 years later.

**The correct response is option D.**

Psychological factors are highly correlated with low back pain; these factors include distress, depressed mood, and somatization, which predict the transition from acute to chronic low back pain.

A minority of patients (about 8%) with acute low back pain will go on to develop chronic low back pain, with disproportionate distress and disability (Carey et al. 2000). The most powerful predictor of chronicity is poor functional status 4 weeks after seeking treatment. In a study of secondary gain, both economic and social rewards were associated with higher levels of disability and depression in patients with chronic nonmalignant back pain (Ciccone et al. 1999). The presence of a depressive disorder has been demonstrated to increase the risk of developing chronic musculoskeletal pain 3 years later. **(p. 831)**

36.4   Using DSM-IV diagnostic criteria for somatoform pain disorder, researchers have estimated the lifetime prevalence of somatoform pain disorder to be

A. 5%.
B. 12%.
C. 17%.
D. 22%.
E. 34%.

**The correct response is option B.**

The lifetime prevalence of somatoform pain disorder (as defined by DSM-III-R [American Psychiatric Association 1987] criteria) in the general population was 34%, with a 6-month prevalence of 17% (Grabe et al. 2003). However, when the DSM-IV (American Psychiatric Association 1994) requirement of significant distress or psychosocial impairment was added to make the diagnosis, the lifetime prevalence was only 12%, and the 6-month prevalence decreased to 5%, with the female-to-male ratio remaining 2:1. **(p. 834)**

36.5   During the first 5 years after the onset of chronic pain, patients are at increased risk of developing new substance use disorders and experiencing additional physical injuries. This risk is highest in patients with a history of

A. Substance abuse or dependence.
B. Childhood physical abuse.
C. Psychiatric comorbidity.
D. Childhood sexual abuse.
E. All of the above.

**The correct response is option E.**

During the first 5 years after the onset of chronic pain, patients are at increased risk for developing new substance use disorders and incurring additional physical injuries (Brown et al. 1996; Savage 1993). This risk is highest in patients with a history of substance abuse or dependence, childhood physical or sexual abuse, and psychiatric comorbidity (Aronoff 2000; Fishbain et al. 1998; Miotto et al. 1996). **(p. 835)**

36.6    Regarding the use of antidepressants to treat pain, which of the following statements is *false*?

A. The selective serotonin reuptake inhibitors (SSRIs) produce weak antinociceptive effects in animal models of acute pain.

B. A study that used number-needed-to-treat (NNT) methodology to compare tricyclic antidepressants (TCAs) with SSRIs found that TCAs and SSRIs were equally effective in treating neuropathic pain.

C. In patients with chronic low back pain without depression, nortriptyline, but not paroxetine, significantly reduced pain intensity.

D. Drugs with noradrenergic activity are often associated with better analgesic effects than are agents with serotonergic activity alone.

E. Randomized, controlled clinical trials have not demonstrated consistent differences in efficacy among the TCAs.

**The correct response is option B.**

Antidepressants, especially TCAs with optimized serum levels, have been found to be the most effective agents for treatment of neuropathic pain, with the majority of clinical trials enrolling patients with postherpetic neuralgia and diabetic peripheral neuropathy.

The SSRIs produce weak antinociceptive effects in animal models of acute pain. In patients with chronic low back pain without depression, nortriptyline or maprotiline, but not paroxetine, significantly reduced pain intensity. Noradrenergic activity is often associated with better analgesic effects than serotonergic activity alone. The relatively noradrenergic antidepressants include amitriptyline, imipramine, doxepin, nortriptyline, desipramine, and maprotiline. Randomized, controlled trials have not demonstrated consistent differences in efficacy among the TCAs. **(pp. 843–844)**

# References

American Psychiatric Association: Diagnostic and Statistical Manual of Mental Disorders, 3rd Edition, Revised. Washington, DC, American Psychiatric Association, 1987

American Psychiatric Association: Diagnostic and Statistical Manual of Mental Disorders, 4th Edition. Washington, DC, American Psychiatric Association, 1994

Aronoff GM: Opioids in chronic pain management: is there a significant risk of addiction? Curr Rev Pain 4:112–121, 2000

Brown RL, Patterson JJ, Rounds LA, et al: Substance use among patients with chronic pain. J Fam Pract 43:152–160, 1996

Carey TS, Garrett JM, Jackman AM: Beyond the good prognosis: examination of an inception cohort of patients with chronic low back pain. Spine 25:115–120, 2000

Ciccone DS, Just N, Bandilla EB: A comparison of economic and social reward in patients with chronic nonmalignant back pain. Psychosom Med 61:552–563, 1999

Fishbain D, Cutler R, Rosomoff H: Comorbid psychiatric disorders in chronic pain patients. Pain Clin 11:79–87, 1998

Grabe HJ, Meyer C, Hapke U, et al: Somatoform pain disorder in the general population. Psychother Psychosom 72:88–94, 2003

Lake AE 3rd, Saper JR: Chronic headache: new advances in treatment strategies. Neurology 59 (suppl 2):S8–S13, 2002

Merskey H, Lindblom U, Mumford JM, et al: Pain terms: a current list with definitions and notes on usage. Pain Suppl 3:S215–S221, 1986

Miotto K, Compton P, Ling W, et al: Diagnosing addictive disease in chronic pain patients. Psychosomatics 37:223–235, 1996

Savage SR: Addiction in the treatment of pain: significance, recognition and management. J Pain Symptom Manage 8:265–278, 1993

Szirmai A: Vestibular disorders in patients with migraine. Eur Arch Otorhinolaryngol Suppl 1:S55–S57, 1997

# C H A P T E R   3 7

# Psychopharmacology

*Select the single best response for each question.*

37.1 Protein binding may be affected by different disease states and may alter the concentrations of administered medications. Which of the following conditions is associated with an increase, rather than a decrease, in protein binding?

A. Cirrhosis.
B. Hypothyroidism.
C. Bacterial pneumonia.
D. Acute pancreatitis.
E. Renal failure.

**The correct response is option B.**

Hypothyroidism may increase protein binding, whereas cirrhosis, bacterial pneumonia, acute pancreatitis, renal failure, surgery, and trauma are associated with decreased protein binding. **(p. 871)**

37.2 The serotonin syndrome is a potentially serious complication of serotonin-active medications. Its psychiatric presentation can include delirium, agitation, anxiety, irritability, euphoria, and restlessness, among other symptoms. Which of the following medications can contribute to the serotonin syndrome through its actions both as a serotonin agonist and as a serotonin reuptake inhibitor?

A. Buspirone.
B. Mirtazapine.
C. Clomipramine.
D. Tramadol.
E. Nefazodone.

**The correct response is option E.**

Nefazodone (as well as trazodone) acts as both a serotonin agonist and a serotonin reuptake inhibitor. Virtually all serotonin potentiators have been associated with the serotonin syndrome. The antidepressant combinations most often implicated are monoamine oxidase inhibitor (MAOI) + tricyclic antidepressant and MAOI + venlafaxine. **(pp. 880–881, Table 37–4)**

37.3 Anticonvulsants have an essential role in contemporary psychopharmacology but are associated with certain worrisome side effects. Among the following anticonvulsants, which is considered to be the most problematic in terms of cognitive side-effect risks?

A. Topiramate.
B. Gabapentin.
C. Lamotrigine.
D. Valproate.
E. Carbamazepine.

**The correct response is option A.**

Among the anticonvulsants most used in psychiatry, topiramate has the highest risk of cognitive side effects, followed by carbamazepine and valproate, lamotrigine, and gabapentin. Insufficient data are available to rank oxcarbazepam and levetiracetam. **(pp. 885, 888)**

37.4   The syndrome of inappropriate antidiuretic hormone (SIADH) results in a euvolemic hyponatremia. Several psychotropic medications are known to induce SIADH, and the psychosomatic medicine physician should monitor fluid and electrolyte status closely in patients taking these agents. Which of the following anticonvulsants has the greatest risk of inducing SIADH?

   A.  Valproate.
   B.  Gabapentin.
   C.  Lamotrigine.
   D.  Oxcarbazepine.
   E.  Topiramate.

**The correct response is option D.**

Oxcarbazepine and carbamazepine frequently cause SIADH, leading to hyponatremia. Carbamazepine-induced hyponatremia has been reported in 6%–36% of patients (McEvoy 2003; van Amelsvoort et al. 1994). Hyponatremia may be more common with oxcarbazepine than with carbamazepine (Asconape 2002). **(p. 886)**

37.5   Clozapine is a revolutionary antipsychotic but has been associated with problematic and sometimes life-threatening medication side effects. Which of the following is *not* true of clozapine-associated cardiac side effects?

   A.  Myocarditis, cardiomyopathy, and heart failure have all been reported.
   B.  Most cases of myocarditis develop between 6 and 12 months after starting treatment.
   C.  Myocarditis has been associated with eosinophilia.
   D.  Cardiomyopathy has most often occurred in patients younger than 50 years.
   E.  Clozapine withdrawal may improve cardiac disease.

**The correct response is option B.**

Eighty-five percent of myocarditis cases develop during the first 2 months of clozapine therapy and may be associated with eosinophilia. Myocarditis and cardiomyopathy have also been associated with chlorpromazine, fluphenazine, risperidone, and haloperidol. **(p. 889)**

37.6   Because of its potential for cardiac conduction problems, which atypical antipsychotic must be avoided in patients receiving drugs with quinidine-like antiarrhythmic properties?

   A.  Clozapine.
   B.  Quetiapine.
   C.  Ziprasidone.
   D.  Risperidone.
   E.  Olanzapine.

**The correct response is option C.**

Low-potency antipsychotics and ziprasidone should be avoided in patients who are taking other drugs with quinidine-like properties. **(p. 890)**

37.7    Which of the following benzodiazepines is eliminated primarily by conjugation and renal excretion, and thus may be *less* problematic in liver disease patients?

   A. Alprazolam.
   B. Clonazepam.
   C. Diazepam.
   D. Oxazepam.
   E. Midazolam.

**The correct response is option D.**

Oxazepam, lorazepam, and temazepam are eliminated primarily by conjugation and renal excretion. **(p. 891)**

37.8    For the agitated patient without oral access, intravenous valproic acid may be a therapeutic option for the psychosomatic medicine physician. Which of the following is *not* true about intravenous valproate?

   A. Intravenous valproic acid (Depacon) was approved by the U.S. Food and Drug Administration (FDA) in 1997.
   B. The medication may be diluted in normal saline.
   C. The maximum infusion rate is 20 mg/minute.
   D. Cardiac monitoring is required.
   E. It is the only mood stabilizer available in parenteral form.

**The correct response is option D.**

The infusion does not require cardiac monitoring and causes no significant risk of orthostatic hypotension.
    Valproic acid can be given in dextrose, saline, or lactated Ringer's solution. The maximum infusion rate is 20 mg/minute, with the dosage reduced in the elderly and in those with organic brain syndromes. **(pp. 897–898)**

# References

Asconape JJ: Some common issues in the use of antiepileptic drugs. Semin Neurol 22:27–39, 2002

McEvoy G (ed): American Hospital Formulary Service (AHFS) Drug Information 2003. Bethesda, MD, American Society of Health-System Pharmacists, 2003

van Amelsvoort T, Bakshi R, Devaux CB, et al: Hyponatremia associated with carbamazepine and oxcarbazepine therapy: a review. Epilepsia 35:181–188, 1994

# CHAPTER 38

# Psychosocial Treatments

*Select the single best response for each question.*

38.1 Group therapy has shown considerable success as an adjunctive treatment for patients with a number of medical illnesses. Patients with which of the following disorders would be good candidates for group therapy?

A. Heart disease.
B. HIV.
C. Breast cancer.
D. A and C.
E. A, B, and C.

**The correct response is option E.**

Group therapy has shown considerable success as an adjunctive treatment for cancer, HIV, heart disease, and other chronic illnesses. Nonetheless, some patients may not feel comfortable in a group setting. For example, patients treated for testicular cancer indicated a preference for individual rather than group psychotherapy (Moynihan et al. 1998). Group therapy may not be the treatment of choice for medically ill patients with severe psychopathology or brain damage. **(p. 926)**

38.2 All of the following are important tasks for group leaders in facilitating discussion among group members *except*

A. Start and end the group on time.
B. Follow the content and not the affect in the room.
C. Respond to problems rather than accumulate unresolved difficulties.
D. Bring group discussions into the room.
E. Make each member feel that his or her problems are as important as anyone else's.

**The correct response is option B.**

Leaders should "follow the affect" in the room rather than the content.

The leader is responsible for starting and ending the group on time and for ensuring that there are few interruptions of the group time. The leader should find a means of addressing problems, thus reducing the helplessness engendered by the problems. Leaders are taught to bring group discussions "into the room" by keeping the focus on interactions occurring among group members rather than directing discussion toward people and events outside the group. Each member should be made to feel that his or her problems are as important as anyone else's problems. **(pp. 927–928)**

38.3 Hypnosis has been found to be effective in treating all of the following clinical situations or medical disorders *except*

A. Acute procedural pain.
B. Irritable bowel syndrome.
C. Traumatic brain injury.
D. Smoking control.
E. Chronic pain.

**The correct response is option C.**

Hypnosis has *not* been found to be effective in the treatment of traumatic brain injury.

According to Patterson and Jensen (2003, p. 495), "randomized, controlled studies with clinical populations indicate that hypnosis has a reliable and significant impact on acute procedural pain and chronic pain conditions." Hypnotic techniques have been shown to effectively reduce cancer pain in adults and procedural pain and other symptoms in children. Hypnosis has also been effective in reducing symptoms in irritable bowel syndrome and asthma and in smoking control. **(pp. 931–932)**

38.4 Psychosocial interventions have been reported to benefit patients with which of the following medical conditions?

A. Cancer.
B. Heart disease.
C. Diabetes.
D. Arthritis.
E. All of the above.

**The correct response is option E.**

Many different types of psychosocial interventions are now available for the medically ill, although evaluation of psychotherapy outcomes has been hampered by enormous variability between studies. Psychosocial interventions appear to benefit patients with cancer, heart disease, diabetes, arthritis, and HIV/AIDS. **(p. 935)**

38.5 Which type of psychosocial intervention, as an adjunct to medical treatment for management of HIV, has most frequently been reported to be effective in reducing distress or psychiatric symptoms?

A. Cognitive-behavioral stress management (CBSM).
B. Hypnosis.
C. Interpersonal psychotherapy (ITP).
D. Brief psychodynamic psychotherapy.
E. Family therapy.

**The correct response is option A.**

Psychosocial interventions have been used as an adjunct to medical treatment and have been shown to benefit emotional health as well as physiological parameters in people with HIV/AIDS. The most commonly effective type of intervention seems to be cognitive-behavioral stress management. **(p. 947, Table 38–6)**

# References

Moynihan C, Bliss JM, Davidson J, et al: Evaluation of adjuvant psychological therapy in patients with testicular cancer: randomised controlled trial. BMJ 316:429–435, 1998

Patterson DR, Jensen MP: Hypnosis and clinical pain. Psychol Bull 129:495–521, 2003

# C H A P T E R  3 9

# Electroconvulsive Therapy

*Select the single best response for each question.*

39.1   Although electroconvulsive therapy (ECT) is generally a well-tolerated procedure from a cardiovascular perspective, certain hemodynamic considerations apply. All of the following statements are true *except*

   A. The barbiturate anesthetic used in ECT increases pulse rate and cardiac output immediately after induction.
   B. After suprathreshold stimulation, the initial parasympathetic phase is followed by a sympathetic phase with tachycardia.
   C. During the seizure, cardiac output increases by 80%.
   D. Increased myocardial workload during ECT may be risky for patients with coronary artery disease and/or congestive heart failure.
   E. Subthreshold electrical stimulation may lead to bradycardia and asystole.

**The correct response is option A.**

The barbiturate anesthetic typically used in ECT increases pulse rate by approximately 25% and decreases cardiac output by 13% immediately after anesthesia. **(p. 958)**

39.2   Similarly to the hemodynamic effects of ECT, there are associated electrocardiogram (ECG) changes. Which of the following statements is *true*?

   A. Sympathetically mediated dysrhythmic ECG changes in ECT include nodal rhythms.
   B. Brief changes in the P-R and QTc intervals may be seen during and immediately following the ECT seizure.
   C. Postseizure premature ventricular contractions (PVCs) are more intense if antimuscarinic premedication is used.
   D. T-wave inversions in ECT generally herald myocardial compromise.
   E. Increased T-wave amplitude during and after the seizure is seen in the majority of patients.

**The correct response is option B.**

Brief, rapidly resolving electrocardiographic changes in the P-R interval, QTc interval, and ST-T wave may be seen during and shortly after the seizure.

Nodal rhythms are parasympathetically mediated ECG changes. Postseizure PVCs are less intense when anticholinergic premedication is used. Transient T-wave inversions can occur in the absence of myocardial compromise. Only 23% of ECT patients showed increased T-wave amplitude. **(p. 959)**

39.3 The depressed patient with chronic atrial fibrillation may benefit from ECT. However, certain precautions are necessary. Which of the following statements is *not* true?

A. Therapeutic anticoagulation should be maintained during the course of ECT.
B. In the patient not receiving chronic anticoagulation, short-term anticoagulation should not be initiated prior to ECT.
C. Transesophageal echocardiography to check for an atrial clot may be desirable.
D. The heart rate should be carefully controlled during ECT.
E. A beta-blocker as premedication may lessen ECT-associated sympathetic stimulation.

**The correct response is option B.**

For the patient who is not receiving chronic anticoagulation, consideration should be given for short-term anticoagulation during the ECT course. **(p. 964)**

39.4 Parkinson's disease is a convenient clinical model for mood and cognitive disorders associated with a neurological illness. Because of the dual comorbidities of depression and dementia frequently encountered in these patients, the use of ECT is subject to some considerations specific for Parkinson's disease. Which of the following statements is *not* true?

A. ECT may improve the motor symptoms of Parkinson's disease.
B. Maintenance ECT treatment may extend clinical response.
C. Acute confusional states following ECT may be minimized by lowering the dose of Parkinson's medication.
D. Due to the severity of depression in these cases, thrice-weekly treatment is typically necessary, even in cognitively impaired patients.
E. Right unilateral or bifrontal electrode placement are preferred.

**The correct response is option D.**

In Parkinson's disease, ECT is recommended twice, versus thrice, weekly with placement of electrodes in the right unilateral or bifrontal area.
Maintenance ECT treatment may extend clinical response, although the benefits need to be balanced against cognitive impairment. **(pp. 968–969)**

39.5 Regarding the use of ECT in depressed patients with comorbid epilepsy, which of the following statements is *true*?

A. With ECT, there is a progressive increase in the seizure threshold and increase in seizure length during a course of treatment.
B. Pre-ECT computed tomography (CT) or magnetic resonance imaging (MRI) of the head should be routinely obtained.
C. Pre-ECT repeated electroencephalogram (EEG) is generally required.
D. The patient's anticonvulsant regimen should be maintained.
E. Hyperventilation before the electrical stimulus may help to produce a seizure.

**The correct response is option E.**

Hyperventilation before the electrical stimulus may produce a seizure.
ECT has anticonvulsant activity, and there is progressive increase in seizure threshold and decrease in seizure length. Imaging of the head or EEG are not needed prior to ECT, unless such testing is indicated as part of the patient's neurological care. Cautious lowering of the patient's anticonvulsant medication dosage is recommended. **(p. 970)**

# C H A P T E R   4 0

# Palliative Care

*Select the single best response for each question.*

40.1 Fully developed model palliative care programs ideally include all of the following components *except*

A. Internet-based services.
B. Intensive care unit.
C. Home care program.
D. Day care program.
E. Bereavement program.

**The correct response is option B.**

Intensive care units are not utilized in palliative care programs.

Fully developed model palliative care programs ideally include all of the following components: 1) a home care program (e.g., hospice program); 2) a hospital-based palliative care consultation service; 3) a day care program or ambulatory care clinic; 4) a palliative care inpatient unit (or dedicated palliative care beds in hospital); 5) a bereavement program; 6) training and research programs; and 7) Internet-based services. It is estimated that there are currently more than 3,000 hospices in the United States and more than 3,000 hospital-based pain and palliative care services. **(p. 980)**

40.2 "Appropriate death" has been defined as

A. Reducing internal conflicts, such as fears about loss of control, as much as possible.
B. Sustaining an individual's personal sense of identity.
C. Enhancing or maintaining critical relationships.
D. Setting and attempting to reach meaningful goals, such as attending a graduation, etc.
E. All of the above.

**The correct response is option E.**

Weisman (1972) described four criteria for what he called an "appropriate death": 1) internal conflicts, such as fears about loss of control, should be reduced as much as possible; 2) the individual's personal sense of identity should be sustained; 3) critical relationships should be enhanced or at least maintained, and conflicts should be resolved, if possible; and 4) the person should be encouraged to set and attempt to reach meaningful goals, even though limited, such as attending a graduation, a wedding, or the birth of a child, as a way to provide a sense of continuity into the future. **(p. 981)**

40.3    Regarding anxiety disorders in terminally ill patients, which of the following statements is *true*?

A.  The prevalence of anxiety disorders among terminally ill cancer patients and AIDS patients is low, in the range of 5%–10%.

B.  Prevalence studies of anxiety, primarily in cancer populations, report a higher prevalence of anxiety alone rather than mixed anxiety and depressive symptoms.

C.  Anxiety in terminally ill patients can occur as an adjustment disorder, a disease or treatment-related condition, or an exacerbation of a preexisting anxiety disorder.

D.  It is important to rapidly taper benzodiazepines and opioids during the terminal phase of illness to minimize the risk of dependence.

E.  None of the above.

**The correct response is option C.**

Anxiety can occur in terminally ill patients as an adjustment disorder, a disease- or treatment-related condition, or an exacerbation of a preexisting anxiety disorder.

Prevalence of anxiety disorders among terminally ill cancer and AIDS patients ranges from 15% to 28%. Prevalence studies of anxiety, primarily in cancer populations, report a higher prevalence of mixed anxiety and depressive symptoms rather than anxiety alone. During the terminal phase of illness, when patients become less alert, there is a tendency to minimize the use of sedating medications. It is important to consider the need to slowly taper benzodiazepines and opioids, which may have been sustained at high doses for extended relief of anxiety or pain, in order to prevent acute withdrawal states. **(p. 983)**


40.4    Factors noted in patients with a desire for hastened death, in contrast to those without this desire, include all of the following *except*

A.  Depression.
B.  More pain.
C.  Pessimistic cognitive style.
D.  Personality disorder.
E.  Less social support.

**The correct response is option D.**

Personality disorders do not seem to increase a desire for hastened death.

Chochinov et al. (1995) found that 45% of terminally ill patients in a palliative care facility acknowledged at least a fleeting desire to die, but these episodes were mostly brief and did not reflect a sustained or committed desire to die. However, 9% reported an unequivocal desire for death to come soon and indicated that they held this desire consistently over time. Among this group, 59% received a diagnosis of depression, compared with a prevalence of 8% in patients who did not endorse a genuine, consistent desire for death. Patients with depression were approximately six to seven times more likely to have a desire for hastened death than patients without depression. Patients with a desire for death were also found to have significantly more pain and less social support than those patients without a desire for death. Both depression and hopelessness, characterized as a pessimistic cognitive style rather than an assessment of one's poor prognosis, appear to be synergistic determinants of desire for hastened death. No significant association with the presence or the intensity of pain was found. **(p. 988)**

40.5 Although words such as *grief*, *mourning*, and *bereavement* are commonly used interchangeably, which of the definitions below is the correct definition for bereavement?

A. State of loss resulting from death.
B. The process of adaptation, including the cultural and social rituals prescribed as accompaniments.
C. The emotional response associated with loss.
D. A pathological outcome involving psychological, social, or physical morbidity.
E. None of the above.

**The correct response is option A.**

Bereavement is the state of loss resulting from death.

Mourning is the process of adaptation, including the cultural and social rituals prescribed as accompaniments. Grief is the emotional response associated with loss. Complicated grief represents a pathological outcome involving psychological, social, or physical morbidity. **(p. 997)**

# References

Chochinov HM, Wilson KG, Enns M, et al: Desire for death in the terminally ill. Am J Psychiatry 152:1185–1191, 1995

Weisman AD: On Dying and Denying: A Psychiatric Study of Terminality. New York, Behavioral Publications, 1972